Introduction to Medical Imaging Management

Bernie Rubenzer, MBA, FAHRA

CRC Press
Taylor & Francis Group
Boca Raton London New York

CRC Press is an imprint of the
Taylor & Francis Group, an **informa** business

CRC Press
Taylor & Francis Group
6000 Broken Sound Parkway NW, Suite 300
Boca Raton, FL 33487-2742

Version Date: 20121120

International Standard Book Number: 978-1-4398-9183-4 (Hardback)

Visit the Taylor & Francis Web site at
http://www.taylorandfrancis.com

and the CRC Press Web site at
http://www.crcpress.com

I dedicate this book to my brother, Dr. Ron Rubenzer. He encouraged me to write, to finish my education, and to stretch myself professionally. He gave me guidance, support, and friendship, and served as my mentor for many years. I owe most of my success to him.

Contents

SECTION II Human Resource Management

SECTION III Operations Management

Preface

Introduction to Medical Imaging Management is designed to be a reference book. In the past, for the most part, people who moved into management positions in medical imaging were chosen because they were the best technologists. The skill set for technologists and supervisors/managers is vastly different. Most management skills in medical imaging were learned through a combination of education and experience.

Even an MBA-prepared person may not be ready to take on imaging management. As an example, when buying a very expensive piece of imaging equipment, this person would not necessarily know the right questions to ask, such as: what is my guaranteed uptime? Is technologist training included?

I have tried to cover all of the important aspects of the business side of imaging. This book is meant to be an overview. It is not meant to be comprehensive in any area discussed. Each area, such as marketing or finance, is its own specialty, and much more specialty material is available for the new manager out in the market.

My hope is that people new to medical imaging management will not be as overwhelmed as many of us "seasoned" managers were when taking on this new role.

Best of luck to all of you in your medical imaging management endeavors!

About the Author

Bernie Rubenzer, MBA, FAHRA, R.T.(R) has been involved in medical imaging for many years. He started his career training as an x-ray technologist in the military, subsequently received a BS in healthcare administration from Western Michigan University in 1987 and an MBA from Keller/DeVry in 1990.

Rubenzer is an author and was a presenter for the American Healthcare Radiology Administrators (AHRA). He is currently a fellow of the AHRA. He has served as a regional president and national board member and committee person for AHRA, in addition to being the president of the Medical Imaging Assembly for the Medical Group Management Association (MGMA). He is also a past president of the Radiology Administrators of Southeast Wisconsin and a committee member of the Radiology Business Management Association (RBMA). He is a member of the American College of Healthcare Executives and the American College of Medical Practice Executives.

Outside of medical imaging, Rubenzer is a member of Mensa.

He is currently the director of imaging for Gila Regional Medical Center in Silver City, New Mexico.

Section I

Introduction

1 Transition to Management

Gayle has been a staff technologist at Pacific Imaging Center for about two years. She has enjoyed her tenure there up to this point. Gayle usually works with several part-time and full-time people, and has a good working relationship with everyone. Two of the other staff members have become her good friends, and Gayle regularly has lunch with them or they stop for a drink after work.

Sally has been Gayle's supervisor since Gayle started. They have worked well together, and Gayle respects her professionalism and fairness. This morning, Sally came in and announced that her husband has taken a job in another city and she will be leaving in three weeks. About an hour later, Gayle received a call from the imaging center administrator, who asked Gayle to come to her office. "As you know, Sally gave her notice this morning. We thought that rather than going through the expensive and time-consuming process of looking outside for her replacement, we would like you to consider taking on this role," the administrator said.

At first, Gayle is quite excited about the prospect. It means a pay increase and will also start to move her along the career ladder. But, after a little bit of thought, Gayle starts to ponder what she is in for in the next several months if she accepts the position. She has spent quite a bit of time working directly with patients and other department staff. Daily interaction and experiences all added to her knowledge, including practical aspects such as how to deal with difficult patients or how to obtain the clinical information the radiologist needs to make a proper diagnosis. Gayle's area of concern has been focused on these types of activities. Now she needs to consider what she will be doing and what she will have to deal with moving into this new role. How will the other people she works with react? What will she experience taking on this new role? What will she need to know? Where does she go to get this knowledge?

SKILL SETS

Traditionally, good technologists were chosen for supervisory positions. Though there can be some transference of skills, the majority of the skill sets necessary for management is not the same as that required for a technologist. In the past, the only way to acquire most of this information was through experience and a wide variety of disconnected formats. This book was designed with this in mind. It will give the reader a good overall picture of the various skill sets necessary to be a successful manager, and shorten the learning curve, which is usually many years.

Higher level focused management training can and should eventually be obtained to understand the topics in this book in greater depth. Undergraduate courses in business and programs such as Master of Business Administration programs are useful in this regard. In addition, focused programs can be found on the various aspects of medical imaging management such as human resources, finance, and others.

WHAT TO EXPECT

In the new managerial position, one of the challenges will be transitioning from team player to team leader. Additionally, managers have a much wider scope of responsibility such as having one or more people reporting to them, and the performance of these employees is the manager's direct responsibility.

Skills in political and cultural influencing, something that may not have been needed in the past position, will be necessary. Since the scope of responsibility has widened, the manager will be put in the position of trying to keep a variety of personalities content and performing at high levels. These challenges will present themselves in a variety of formats. The manager may have to convince the radiologists that they do not necessarily need the latest and greatest magnetic resonance imaging (MRI) scanner (at a cost of several million dollars) so the hospital's upper management will stay within budget. A very important managerial soft skill is influencing. Just as in the outside world, awareness of different personalities is paramount to being successful.

One of the most difficult issues to deal with is the interaction with former peers. After working side by side with them for some time, now the job calls for leading these same people. It can be a very uncomfortable position to be in at first. Much will depend on how it is handled.

Former peers may be envious or angry for being overlooked and may react in a variety of ways. One of the biggest mistakes a new manager can make is to act as if nothing has changed. Of course it has. A manager typically cannot be as informal in their interactions as in past positions. One main role as a manager is to ensure cooperation, and this may not be easy if a former peer is harboring ill feelings because of the new position. In addition, as more experience is gained in the new role, it is possible to be accused of favoritism—treating one employee better than others—especially if that former peer was a close friend.

Managers sometimes report to someone that they may not have had much contact with in the past. This relationship will now be much more direct, as it will probably be necessary to interact for some reason on a daily basis. Being part of the management team will also change a person's associations. There will be much more contact with other area managers, vendors, referring physicians, and another universe of people that they have never met before.

MOTIVATION

One method to help in understanding human needs is the theory put forth by Abraham Maslow, an eminent psychologist of the early 1940s. He proposed five levels of needs: (1) physiological, (2) safety, (3) love, (4) esteem, and (5) self-actualization (Graphic 1.1).

1. Physiological needs. These are the most basic physical needs, which include food, shelter, clothing, and self-preservation.
2. Safety needs. These are the needs associated with physical safety and emotional needs, which includes avoiding violence and threats.
3. Love needs. Once the basic needs are taken care of, humans look for love, friendship, and affection.
4. Esteem needs. After social needs are met, people focus on self-respect, status, reputation, recognition, and self-confidence.
5. Self-actualization needs. The highest level of need is self fulfillment: the need to develop to the fullest potential, to become the best one is capable of being.

People tend to be at different levels in this hierarchy at different times of their lives. Understanding these needs will help the manager ascertain what approaches need to be taken under certain circumstances. Typically, the esteem and self-actualization levels are most prominent in the work environment. By appealing to these needs, people can be motivated to produce their best work. In the course of this process, in order to create the most efficient and fulfilling work environment, it is incumbent upon the manager to create the environment where these needs can be met.

Another theory in motivation is postulated by Frederick Herzberg in what he calls "needs-based theory." The theory states two motivational aspects: motivating factors and hygiene factors.

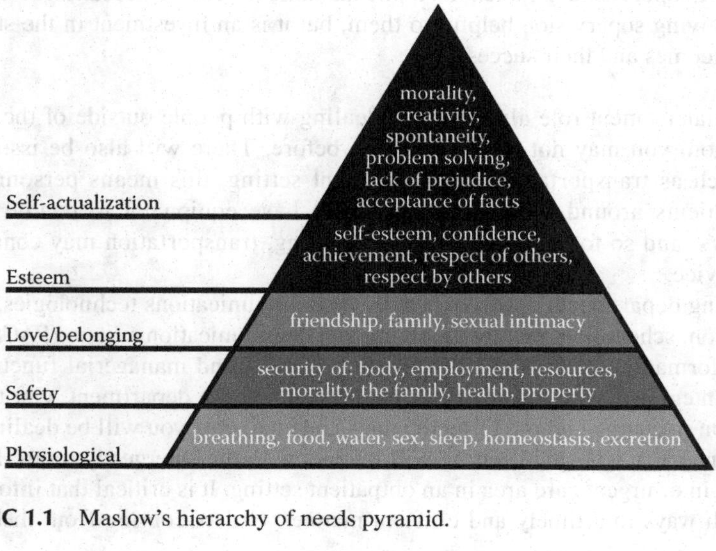

GRAPHIC 1.1 Maslow's hierarchy of needs pyramid.

It is surprising to learn that people's top motivation is not money. According to Herzberg, hygiene factors are lower level needs, such as pay, job security, work relationships, management, and company policies. Motivating factors are achievement, recognition, responsibility, advancement, and growth.

Experts concur that the number one reason people leave their jobs is a poor relationship with their immediate supervisor.

PERSONNEL BASICS

One of the first tasks to tackle is to create an environment of mutual trust and cooperation. Keep in mind what it was like to be a staff person, and this should not be difficult. However, there are some key points here to remember:

- Allow enough time, at least a few months, to assess the department's situation. It is now necessary to view daily activities on a much more global basis.
- Do not try to make a lot of changes immediately. Even if it becomes clear that some things need attention, if they are not urgent, it is better to make changes slowly. When possible, get the staff involved in these changes. It will make them more comfortable with the process while simultaneously promoting buy-in from them.
- Always give praise in public, when possible. Conversely, discipline in private.
- Keep a log on each staff member and notate positive and negative occurrences, which will be used later in performance evaluations.
- Trust the staff's skills. If a previous position required working side by side with staff members, this should have given a fairly good perception of their skill level. If the previous position did not require working side by side with staff members, a few months of observation should provide insight into their skill level.
- Give supervision. People look to the manager to provide guidance. Not only is giving supervision helpful to them, but it is an investment in the staff's outcomes and their success.

The management role also requires dealing with people outside of the department whom you may not have dealt with before. There will also be issues with areas such as transportation. In an inpatient setting, this means personnel who move patients around. Does the department have equipment to handle oxygen tanks, IVs, and so forth? In an outpatient setting, transportation may consist of a valet service.

Imaging departments now rely heavily on communications technologies. Patient registration, scheduling, picture archiving and communication system (PACS), radiology information systems (RIS), and other clerical and managerial functions are heavily integrated with the IT (information technology) department. Get to know the person in charge and the IT technicians and engineers you will be dealing with.

A manager in a hospital setting will interact with the emergency room (ER) and the walk-in or urgent care area in an outpatient setting. It is critical that information flow both ways in a timely and efficient manner. Orders coming from these areas need to be top on the priority list. It is also paramount that communication between these areas and imaging be thorough and efficient. As an example of the importance of this fact, many lawsuits have involved an ER or urgent care physician's initial medical imaging diagnosis differing from that of the radiologist. If the radiologist's differing interpretation is not communicated to the ER or urgent care, patient outcomes can be severely affected.

The medical imaging department must also ensure that communications with the nursing staff are efficient and accurate. Orders for exams and patient clinical information must be confirmed. Results must be delivered to the proper places in a timely manner.

Typically, the imaging department manager will be required to be on the facility's quality assurance committee. This involvement will help raise awareness of information flow though the facility, along with issues in other areas. It all helps to build a knowledge base that will help the manager make better decisions concerning the imaging department.

Think through the processes involved in the registration, scheduling, ordering of studies, performance of studies, returning results, and archiving studies to get an idea of how the required responsibilities are different now. The best way to start is with some management basics.

Some basic tenets are as follows:

- Make sure basic tasks are done.
- Ensure that people have adequate time and materials to perform their jobs effectively.
- Learn team-building skills. The job will be easier and less problematic if everyone is on the same page, going in the same direction.
- Learn to understand group dynamics. This coincides with team building and will provide insight on how to be an effective leader.
- Understand that your former peers may have formed relationships with your superiors. Although the term *office politics* may have a negative connotation, understanding human relationships can be very helpful in the management role.

After acquiring management skills, it will be beneficial to move on to obtaining leadership skills.

LEADERSHIP STYLES

There are many leadership style theories. The bottom line is that leadership requires the use of power. Employees react differently to the type and use of power.

One theory includes five levels of power: (1) legitimate power, (2) reward power, (3) coercive power, (4) expert power, and (5) referent power. The manager may have one or a combination of these powers depending on the organization.

1. Legitimate power is the authority a manager has because of his or her title and position. This manager may have a wide variety of duties. The organization bestows the ability to carry out these duties.

2. Reward power is the potential for a manager to reward in a variety of ways. This can be through pay raises, increase in responsibility, and verbal or written praise.
3. Coercive power is the ability to use a variety of methods for punishment. These methods can range from verbal reprimands to loss of pay, status, and the job itself. Use of this power usually results in negative outcomes.
4. Expert power comprises the manager's knowledge, skills, and expertise. Typically, this is the first level of power used by a technologist who has recently been promoted to manager. In this situation, the technologist usually possesses most of the technical skills needed to perform in an imaging department. This enables him or her to assess and coach others on the technologist level.
5. Referent power is typically used to describe the authority a manager has by virtue of gaining the respect, admiration, and loyalty of his or her employees.

By understanding the different power levels, the manager can understand that leadership in the imaging area is usually a blending of the different types of power. As management experience is obtained, there is a shift from expert power to a combination of the other forms of power.

GENERATIONAL DIFFERENCES

There may be people from many different generations working in the same environment. It is important to understand what their needs, differences, and motivators are.

The first category is called the *matures*. These are people born before about 1946.

The second category is called the *baby boomers*. This category comprises those born between 1946 and 1965.

The third category is *Gen Xers*, born between 1965 and 1976.

The last category is called the *millennials*, who were born between 1977 and 1998.

Chart 1.1 best describes who these people are and what their work needs are.

Engage Me

To Engage Matures	To Engage Baby Boomers
Managers Should... • Take care not to "overdo" recognition, especially for simply doing what is expected. • Be open to alternative schedules - Matures are now typically working because they want to, not because they have to. Retaining them may require flexibility. • Understand and recognize the importance of teamwork - Matures believe the group is more powerful and more important than the individual.	**Managers Should...** • Adopt a "get it done" and "whatever it takes" attitude. • Be visible and active in the workplace - Boomers value "face time" and do not want to be managed from afar. • Demonstrate how you have earned your leadership role. • Have first-hand knowledge of subordinate's work, preferably having done the same job at some point.
Communications Should... • Be spoken and written, this is particularly important for messages that impact the company or their work. • Use traditional formats - text-messaging terms are considered rude and indecipherable. • Come from authority figures in the company - those that have tenure. • Clearly communicate what is needed from them and their teammates.	**Communications Should...** • Highlight team goals, accomplishments, and celebrations. • Focus on team goals, preferably posted in public places where everyone can be reminded of them. • Avoid text-messaging abbreviations. • Demonstrate understanding of stated team goals and be focused on helping the team towards those goals. • Be delivered in person where possible. Email is secondary.
The Corporate Culture Should... • Allow Matures to feel confident and able regarding technology - don't expect mastery without proper training. • Operate under clear rules and expectations, with any changes properly communicated to all. • Provide opportunities to stay in touch with changing expectations, particularly technological skills. • Value their Institutional Wisdom. Call upon Matures for guidance and opinion when appropriate - they are superb teachers.	**The Corporate Culture Should...** • Offer the tools Boomers need to do the job better, more quickly, more thoroughly, etc. • Promote visibility of bosses and workplace peers - "face time" matters. • Acknowledge both individuals and teams who have achieved their goals. • Promote collaborative meetings where everyone can provide input as desired. • Allow Boomers time to anticipate and prepare for change.
Training Programs Should... • Be immediately and clearly relevant. • Use their time wisely. • Invite discussion throughout the training, including how the training will help and its implications on their work. • Provide insights into their workplace peers or clients / customers that they didn't have already. • Be delivered by someone with "earned" authority, not someone who could be their grandchild (unless it is technology skills training).	**Training Programs Should...** • Keep Boomers up-to-date and competitive in a quickly changing and evolving workplace. • Allow all levels of technology skills to learn without feeling inferior or intimidated - pre-evaluate skills, don't assume. • Be participatory and interactive, allowing for deliberation and discussion versus one-way instruction. Ask them more questions than they ask you. • Create realistic examples to utilize in the learning process.
Rewards & Recognition Should... • Celebrate the efforts of the whole team, not any single individual. • Be genuine and sincere. Nothing beats a handshake and a personal "Thank you" from the boss. • Recognize true achievements, not simply rewards for doing the job.	**Rewards & Recognition Should...** • Celebrate the individual as well as the team. • Be public and/or able to be displayed - trophies, plaques, lapel pins, etc. are valued by the Boomer. • Encourage celebrations within the team as well as company-wide acknowledgements.

CHART 1.1 Generational matrix. (From Cam Marston, GenerationalInsights.com. With permission.) (continued)

Matching generational preferences with tactics to help each employee reach his full potential.	
To Engage Gen Xers	**To Engage Millennials**
Managers Should... • Honor commitments at all cost. Gen Xers place a high value on reliability. • Recognize that work does not equal life - celebrate Xers' hobbies or passions in addition to their work skills. • Allow for flexibility and negotiate schedules when needed. • Regularly review individual goals and team goals and the individual's role on the team. • Revisit deadlines as needed.	**Managers Should...** • Have a sincere interest in the individual - spend time with them and get to know their goals and personalities. • Offer and commit to develop new, valuable, and relevant skills in their employees. • Recognize that work does not equal life - have fun. • Offer scheduling flexibility with negotiations (Like Gen X). • Articulate how working for you will help them achieve their personal goals while achieving the company goals at the same time.
Communications Should... • Get straight to the point - Gen Xers loathe fluff. • Be consistent and supported with actions as well as words. The company must walk their talk every day. • Be infrequent. "Official Corporate Communications" should be saved for the critical messages. Most communication should be individualized and delivered personally. • Email is usually the preferred method of communication followed by interpersonal, face-to-face conversation.	**Communications Should...** • Outline the steps needed to achieve a goal. • Establish "checkpoints" along the way to document progress towards goals and provide frequent feedback. • Celebrate individual contributions to team goals where possible. • Be positive. When giving criticism be prepared with a 3:1 positive to negative ratio - three compliments for every one reprimand.
The Corporate Culture Should... • Trust the employee's time management skills - check in regularly but not frequently. • Allow them to get their work done without interference or unnecessary interruptions. Leave them alone when they're focused on their tasks. • Seek their input frequently on what you can do to "to make things better, easier or quicker?" • Respond to their requests with actions and results.	**The Corporate Culture Should...** • Ask "What have you learned today? Anything you think I need to know?" • Avoid strict hierarchy/chains of command; egalitarian approach is preferred. • Seek input from everyone, not just leaders, managers, supervisors, etc. • Encourage optional social activities that are open to all employees and are held outside the office, after hours - adopt and develop an employee Social Calendar. • Give credit to individuals for their ideas and involvement.
Training Programs Should... • Address the employee's career goals - ask "What skills do you need to get where you want to go?" • Be flexible and numerous - Gen Xers want information and choices. • Demonstrate commitment to the Gen Xer mantra to "work smarter not harder." • Include leaders and peers - demonstrating management's commitment to the training as a valuable use of time. • Promote new ideas on how to "get things done."	**Training Programs Should...** • Involve the whole group, where practical. • Clearly identify how they'll benefit from learning this information both at this job and beyond. • Be interactive and fun. • Allow everyone to take a role in some part of the teaching process.
Rewards & Recognition Should... • Offer variety. Allow Gen Xers to choose from a list of reward options with roughly equal values. • Express gratitude for the individual's contribution in private, Xers don't want a fuss for doing their jobs. • Honor commitments to goals that are solid and achievable - don't keep upping the ante or you will lose trust.	**Rewards & Recognition Should...** • Offer options, similar to Gen X needs. Millennials cherish their individuality. • Be celebrated publicly, in front of the team and/or visible to the customer where appropriate (lapel pin, etc). • Offer special "top performer" learning opportunities to reward initiative and help propel employees toward their future goals. • Happen during the work day - validate the reward by celebrating on company time.

CHART 1.1 (continued) Generational matrix. (From Cam Marston, GenerationalInsights.com. With permission.)

2 Management Basics and Skills

COMMUNICATION

The very first skills to learn as a new manager are communication skills. Listening skills are crucial to communication. There are a few accepted methods to improve listening skills. One is to *paraphrase* or repeat the speaker's ideas in your own words. This assures the speaker and listener that ideas are communicated and understood clearly. It is also helpful to repeat key points to assure the speaker that she has been understood by the listener.

The manager will become aware of myriad reasons on a daily basis for clear communication. From upper management's perspective, it will ensure that information from upper management is communicated to the caregivers. It will help to guide all department personnel so that everyone is going in the same direction as the facility's strategic plans and goals. From a staff perspective, good communication will ensure that information from staff is analyzed, digested, and communicated upward. When this loop is in place, staff members feel that their ideas and contributions are valued. The most important aspect of communication in the department is ensuring that patient concerns and care issues are communicated. As a technologist, the manager realizes how important clinical information is for other staff, radiologists, referring physicians, and the various clerical areas involved in care. Clinical history, previous contrast reactions, and previous exams results are just some examples. It is the manager's duty to ensure that lines of communication remain open and clear.

CONFLICT MANAGEMENT

One of the most difficult duties the new manager will have is that of conflict management. Conflict arises from many sources in a busy, highly charged environment. Some problem sources can result from unclear or nonexistent communications. Another source is the degree of involvement a person has in a situation. If people involved do not take part in the process or do so only to a limited degree, they may not fully understand their particular role and its importance.

Personality can be another source of conflict. If employees feel that they are unjustly treated or compensated or that management is not listening to them, they can possess a negative attitude, which often leads to conflict. Occasionally individuals will avoid taking responsibility for a variety of reasons.

A manager's insight is helpful in conflict management. One good method is to attempt to understand the perspective of those involved. Their priorities might be different. This can also be thought of as having one's own agenda.

The material following will help to understand how a person thinks.

Brain Scan: A Five-Minute Exercise

I have half a mind to...
This is a no-brainer...
He is so scatterbrained...
If I only had a brain...

Some of the characteristics that correspond to left- or right-brain thinking styles are listed in the Brain Scan table below. Of course, we always use more than half of our brain when thinking, just as we actually use more than one hand (even back muscles) when we pick up a soda to drink.

How to do your own brain scan:

- Casually read each left-brain/right-brain style choice.
- Circle the one that seems more like you.
- It is OK to circle corresponding opposites if both describe you.
- Add the column totals (write L = [left brain column total]; R = [right brain]).
- The column (left or right) with more items circled suggests your tendency or thinking style (left or right brain).
- Learn to compromise and use both sides of your brain.

At home it is better to be happy than right; at work it is better to be right than happy.

The only adult's mind you can really change is your own. If you are constantly in a state of agitation because everyone else seems scatterbrained, you might consider consciously trying to change your mind. Using the Brain Scan below, you may wish to take a couple of the items that you feel you can't give up (which you are "urgently addicted" to) and try to change them.

Brain Scan (Circle characteristics more like you.)

LEFT BRAIN	RIGHT BRAIN
Early bird	Night owl
Analytical (breaks things down)	Analogical (makes connections)
Prefer clarity	Prefer vagueness
Prefer correct answer	Seek alternative responses
Doer	Dreamer
Exactness and precision desired	Tend to exaggerate
Structured, forced	Unstructured, free
Intellectual	Artistic
Test ideas	Make ideas

Brain Scan (Circle characteristics more like you.) (continued)

LEFT BRAIN	RIGHT BRAIN
Serious	Jokester
Logical	Intuitive
Motivated by external rewards	Motivated by satisfaction
Focused, narrow	Nebulous, diffuse
Makes order out of chaos	Makes chaos out of order
Opinionated	Open minded
Planned	Directionless
Asks factual questions (what, when, who, etc.)	Ask speculative questions (what if, why not)
Rule maker	Rule breaker/bender
Interested in science fact and fiction	Interested in science
By the clock (lunch is always at noon)	Timeless (lunch is "whenever" you are hungry)
Uptight	Uninhibited
Verbal	Visual
Task oriented	Idea oriented
Enjoy complicated	Keep it simple
Astronomy buff	Astrology fan
Loathes surprises	Loves surprises
Total your left and right brain	
Column descriptors ______ L's	Column descriptors ______ R's

Source: Courtesy of D. Oetjen, Conflict Management. doetjen@mail.ucf.edu. With permission.

This exercise will give you an idea of how different personalities operate.

Different interactions take place in the imaging department: staff to staff, staff to radiologists, staff to referring physicians, radiologists to referring physicians, and radiologists to administration are some examples. If the manager thinks about these different situations and what the individual's needs are at that particular time, the manager can better understand how conflict has arisen and some possible solutions.

Although conflict can negatively affect productivity and morale, not all conflict is bad. In fact, conflict is considered functional, rather than dysfunctional, when it helps the organization reach its goals, according to Dawn Oetjen, PhD, associate professor, and Reid Oetjen, PhD, assistant professor, both of the College of Health and Public Affairs, University of Central Florida, Orlando. "By talking about differences openly, we learn and grow and interact effectively," Dawn Oetjen said.[1]

Persuasion is a useful tool in dealing with conflict. Here are some suggestions from Dawn Oetjen:[2]

Only after you understand the other party's motivators and perceptions should you share your viewpoint. Start with your perception of the facts: "Here's how I see it … "

Next, make recommendations for action and state your justification. This could sound like, "I recommend that we … What I'm basing my opinion on is … "

At this stage, it's appropriate to communicate your values and goals. People can't read your mind, so it's up to you to make your needs known. You might say,

"I think you know I feel strongly about … , and that's why I want to … "

"Here's what I hope comes out of this. I think we agree on … "

At this point, you may still be at odds with the other party. Speculate on the reasons for the difference and invite response. Words that prompt exploration and discussion are as follows:

"Why do you think we have such different views?"

"You seem to want a different outcome. Can we talk about why we disagree?"

Ways to Avoid Conflict

One major method of avoiding conflict is to attempt to align priorities and goals. For example, if the patient is where focus is centered, effort will be placed to do what is best for the patient and conflict will not arise as easily. Another way is to ensure clear expectations. The best time to set expectations is during the initial orientation process. These should be defined in the *job description* as well as in an *orientation checklist*. Job descriptions will be discussed in Chapter 4, and orientation checklist will be covered in Chapter 5.

Negotiation

Another vital set of skills for the new manager is negotiation skills. These particular skills are used in many places on almost a daily basis. Some examples of where negotiation skills are necessary are benefits and salary for new hires during the hiring process, annual increases and work assignments with existing employees, collaboration with other departments for a variety of reasons, and of particular importance is negotiation interaction with vendors—equipment vendors, suppliers, service contractors, and others.

Various approaches can be used in negotiation, depending on the people involved. There is give and take to various degrees.

"It's all about me." This is probably the worst approach to negotiation. The negotiator in this situation has only her interest at heart and makes no concessions to the other party. Unless one party has absolutely no choice or is in such a position that they do not need to be flexible (by virtue of title, bullying, etc.) this approach should be avoided. The results of this approach are usually not very satisfactory.

"It's all about you." This can happen when one of the parties is so concerned with pleasing the other that they neglect to keep their own best interests in mind. This is also not a very good negotiating tactic as there is one winner and one loser.

"I don't really want to deal with this." This attitude can be held by one or both parties. This happens when one or both do not want to tackle the negotiation—they would rather put it off or not deal with it at all. It is obvious that no one's needs are served in this case.

"You take some and I'll take some." This approach is kind of a meeting in the middle. Both parties receive some degree of satisfaction with the results. Although the outcome is good, it is not the best.

"Maybe we can both have more" (*synergistic*). This is the best-case scenario. This results when the parties involved work together and the result is better than both had expected.

In planning for negotiation, the manager should decide how much he is willing to concede, and how much he *must* gain versus how much he would *like to* gain. Try to figure out the same for the other parties involved. This will give the manager better insight into the process and possible results.

There are many permutations and different combinations of these scenarios. Having the basic knowledge and doing the homework ahead of time when possible will lead to the best possible outcome.

DELEGATION

The ability to delegate will help the new manager make the best use of her time. The particular skill sets of individuals can be utilized. As an example, if a particular individual is better at data gathering than the manager, that person should be used for that task.

Delegation has changed much in the past 50 years. In the past, delegation was done by direct order or assignment. Dealing with people as individuals rather than commodities in recent times has enabled much higher levels of performance

To begin, the manager should make a list of old versus new skills necessary in delegation.

- Whenever possible, when delegating work, give the person a whole task to do. (If you can't give the employee a whole task, make sure he understands the overall purpose of the project or task. If possible, connect him to the group that is managing or planning the work. Staff members contribute most effectively when they are aware of the big picture.)
- Make sure the staff person understands exactly what you want her to do. Ask questions, watch the work being performed, or have the employee give you feedback to make sure your instructions were understood.
- If you have a picture of what a successful outcome or output will look like, share your picture with the staff person. You want to make the person right. You don't want to fool the person to whom you delegate authority for a task into believing that any outcome will do, unless you really feel that way.
- Identify the key points of the project or dates when you want feedback about progress. This is a critical path that provides you with the feedback you need without causing you to micromanage your direct report or team. You need assurance that the delegated task or project is on track. You also need the opportunity to influence the project's direction and the team or individual's decisions.

- Identify the measurements or the outcome you will use to determine that the project was successfully completed. (This will make performance development planning more measurable and less subjective, too.)
- Determine, in advance, how you will thank and reward the staff person for the successful completion of the task or project you delegated.

Successful delegation of authority as a leadership style takes time and energy, but it's worth the time and energy to help employee involvement and employee empowerment succeed as a leadership style. It's worth the time and energy to help employees succeed, develop, and meet your expectations. You build the employees' self-confidence, and people who feel successful usually are successful.

Delegation as a Leadership Style

Tips for Effective Delegation

By Susan M. Heathfield[3]

Delegation allows the manager to focus their attention on higher level tasks— not get bogged down with daily details. Decide what can be delegated. When thinking through the process, it is advisable to document those tasks that can be delegated, those that should be delegated, and those that should be performed directly by the manager. This will vary by the people involved and the tasks to be performed. There may be situations where the manager's immediate superior prefers that she or he perform a task rather than a staff person, even though it may be well within the staff member's skills to perform that task.

As part of the delegation process, it is important to recognize those helping with the delegated task. It gives them a sense of appreciation and involvement. Trust in the delegate is important. To complete the task in the most efficient and effective manner, the manager must give authority to complete the task.

Deadlines for portions of the project should be set. They should be reachable and enough time should be allotted.

The manager should be sure to monitor, document, and evaluate what the designee is doing. In the end, the manager is ultimately responsible for the outcome.

PRIORITIZING/ORGANIZATION

One of the difficulties the new manager will encounter is the juggling act between patient and physician demand, and staff and upper management wishes. There is only so much energy that can be devoted to any one task at a given time. Much of the time, however, the manager will be tackling multiple tasks at the same time. How is this best managed?

First of all, priorities must be set. While there are tasks that require immediate attention (putting out fires), the manager should not spend their entire day moving from one fire to another.

One way to approach prioritizing is to construct a to-do list each morning. Look at the tasks that require attention and rank them, putting the *high-impact/high-visibility* tasks first. High-impact tasks are those that have the most immediate or far-reaching consequences. As an example, patient-focused tasks that have an effect on care would be high impact. High-visibility tasks are those that would get the attention of upper management. An example is a first budget draft that is due by the end of the week.

It is also advisable to tackle the most difficult tasks first. Although it is a natural tendency to put these types of tasks off because they may be uncomfortable, people's energy level is usually higher first thing in the morning rather than, say, right after lunch.

A skill that should be mastered after learning to prioritize is *time management.* This will be covered in a later section.

PRESENTATION SKILLS

Presentation skills are a must for the new manager. These skills will be used for staff meetings, budget presentations, and facility committee involvement to groups such as physician administrators, board for joint ventures, and community presentations—health fairs, media interaction (newspapers, TV, etc.), and others.

There are typically three purposes for a presentation: to influence, to inform, and to convince. It is necessary to know the group you are presenting to in order to correctly apply the skills needed to achieve the objectives of your presentation.

The four basic needs an audience wants to have met were presented by Dr. David Campbell, an award-winning speaker with the Center for Creative Leadership (coauthor of the Campbell Strong Interest Inventory). He emphasized the four basic components that successful workshop presenters need to have:

1. Credentials/accomplishments of the presenters (degrees, associations, publications).
2. Content: "What to do tomorrow" activities or information.
3. Entertainment: Relevant humor and stories. Your presentation is competing with popular media as a baseline expectation. Use graphics and visual media when possible.
4. Resourcefulness of speaker to recover in case things go wrong (e.g., equipment failure).

Doing a Needs Assessment: What Is Your Training Bull's-Eye?

Ask training needs assessment questions. Are the training needs process or outcome based?

Example of process goal: Train teachers about test-taking strategies and have students learn test-taking skills as part of the curriculum.

Example of outcome goal: Test scores will improve. Find out what results (goals) are most highly rewarded in the system.

What goals/results receive recognition?

Spend 20% of the workshop finding out what the participants need. Write out workshop activities as they connect with the identified needs the workshop is to meet.

Single-factor emphasis: Most participants will remember only one simple fact one year after the workshop. Define, highlight, and emphasize the most important thing to remember from the workshop.

Bells and Whistles

Here are eight tips to use in trying not to bore or baffle your audience. You are competing with sophisticated mass media (TV, radio). Learn from these media in terms of simplicity, colorfulness, and appeal of your presentation.

- Use color where possible.
- Use music where possible.
- All overheads should be legible. (You should be able to read the material from a five-foot distance without projection.)
- Handouts should match overheads (where possible).
- Limit key points to five or seven maximum.
- Give people a choice to participate in simulations.
- Use banners/props where appropriate.
- Provide snacks.

Content Development: Seven Strategies to Make Sure You Are on Target

1. Incentive (Remember WII-FM—What's in it for me?) What will your participants gain personally and/or professionally from your talk?
2. E. F. Hutton statement ("Wow! I didn't know that" statements). Make bold and truthful statements.
3. Speak their language. Use the audience's language. People can only absorb five to seven new facts at a time. Know your audience.
4. Remember the 7-7 rule. Stick to seven major points; repeat the main points seven times (in different forms).
5. Take hourly breaks if possible. The average adult attention span is 45 minutes.
6. Did we hit the bull's-eye? Or was there good ROI—return on investment? For the investment (time/money), what measurable, positive change has been realized? Ask your participants what single change they will make as the result of the workshop. How will this change be documented? (It can be a process or outcome change.)
7. Attention-getter notes from the audience. Distribute two or three index cards to each participant. Tell them ahead of time that you will randomly ask them to write down whatever they are thinking about at a particular moment during your talk. Have each participant do this individually, and anonymously.

The manager may wish to delay telling the audience they don't have to put their names on the cards till right before they turn in their cards. This will increase their attention span. (This is to your attention-getting ability, not their listening skills.) Have them pass in the cards (with no identification) right after you ask them to write down their predominant thought at that moment. Review these cards, and see how many bull's-eyes you were hitting with your talk. Turn up the volume for points not getting through by reducing the number of points or increasing the interest level of your points.

Presenter Preparation: Tips to Guarantee Success

1. Don't sweat (while presenting).
2. Sweat while preparing. Ten to one ratio of preparation to presentation time is typical. (It takes 10 hours of preparation for an hour of good presentation.) This includes needs assessment, product development, and practice.
3. Attitude affirmation. Repeat to yourself, "I know that I know this material," to build your confidence. You will always know a little more than your audience (at least new jokes). Smile and say to yourself and then to your audience, "I'm glad to be here," (whether you are or not, fake it till you make it). Smiling will make your audience think you're smart. Find one friendly face in the audience.
4. "Tattoo your speech on your brain."
5. Use the rule of 7. Go through your talk at least seven times. Practice once to a live audience (of one) sitting at the back of the room or tape record your speech. Make sure your practice audience feigns boredom and distraction so you are not upset when it happens in real life. Have your guinea pig audience sit at least 20 feet away from you so you learn to project your voice.
6. Double the amount of enthusiasm you speak with normally and slow down your pace.
7. Practice the main points of your speech right before you go to sleep. This will solidify it in your memory.
8. Drink a warm (decaffeinated) drink right before you talk. It will relax you and your voice. Take three or four slow, deep breaths, belly breathing if you can. Breathe in through your nose, and exhale from your mouth.
9. Use cue cards and technology, but don't depend on them entirely.

Have your major points memorized. TV personalities use kindergarten-letter-sized type on their notes. Probably a 20-point font size would be helpful. Also, you can even put breathing/pause marks in your notes so you don't talk too fast under stress. A breathing mark in your notes is simply a slash. Professional speakers use breathing marks in their notes. Remember: *Practice makes permanent*.

Putting It All Together with the Step-by-Step Workshop Worksheet Checklist (Check items as they apply. See text for explanation of each item.)

Needs Assessment: What Is Your Training Bull's-Eye?

FOUR BASIC NEEDS

- Credentials of presenters
- Content "What to do tomorrow" based on knowledge
- Entertainment—humor that is relevant
- Resourcefulness to recover (Plan B if Plan A doesn't work)

Other Considerations

- Process or outcome (end point) goals of training defined
- Rewarded results identified and used as goals for training
- Twenty percent of workshop time used in participant identification of needs
- Workshop activities connect with identified goals/needs
- Single fact to be remembered is defined and highlighted

BELLS AND WHISTLES

- Color used where possible
- Music used where possible
- Overheads all legible
- Handouts match overheads (where appropriate)
- Limit key points to five to seven items
- Give people choice in simulations
- Props, posters used
- Edibles

CONTENT DEVELOPMENT

- WII-FM (What's in it for me?) Incentives for participants
- E. F. Hutton, truthful statements
- Speak their language (Know your audience)
- 7-7 rule: (Limit of seven major points; repeat main points seven times)
- Hourly breaks (if possible)
- Was training bull's-eye hit? Use an outcome measure (before/after quiz results on topic)
- Attention-getter notes. Randomly ask all participants to write down what they are thinking during the talk on index cards given out earlier. No identification is needed on cards submitted. Use feedback to improve your message and/or delivery.

PRESENTER PREPARATION

- Expect 10 hours of preparation for 1 hour of initial presentation.

- Practice attitude affirmation to build self-confidence (I know that I know this material).
- Smile and say, “I’m glad to be here.” Think of friends in audience.
- Go through talk seven times prior to speech.
- Double the amount of enthusiasm when you speak.
- Slow down your rate of speech.
- Practice your speech the night before with your warm-up audience faking boredom.
- Drink a warm decaffeinated drink right before your talk.
- Take a few deep breaths.
- Use cue cards but memorize key points.

BODY LANGUAGE

Body language, when used properly, will enhance a presentation. A confident, enthusiastic presentation can be bolstered by correct posture and movement.

MOTIVATING

The basics of motivation were covered in Chapter 1 in the discussion of Maslow’s hierarchy of needs. The bottom line is that only the self can motivate. The best way to help to motivate others is to be an example as a manager. If staff observes the manager as conscientious, hard working, and dedicated, they understand that the same should be expected of them.

HERZBERG’S MOTIVATION-HYGIENE THEORY

Frederick Herzberg performed studies to determine which factors in an employee’s work environment caused satisfaction or dissatisfaction. He published his findings in the 1959 book *The Motivation to Work*. The studies included interviews in which employees were asked what pleased and displeased them about their work. Herzberg found that the factors causing job satisfaction (and presumably motivation) were different from those causing job dissatisfaction. He developed the *motivation-hygiene* theory to explain these results. He called the satisfiers *motivators* and the dissatisfiers *hygiene factors*, using the term *hygiene* in the sense that these are considered maintenance factors that are necessary to avoid dissatisfaction but that by themselves do not provide satisfaction. The following table presents the top six factors causing dissatisfaction and the top six factors causing satisfaction, listed in the order of higher to lower importance.

Leading to Dissatisfaction	Leading to Satisfaction
Company policy	Achievement
Supervision	Recognition
Relationship with boss	Work itself
Work conditions	Responsibility
Salary	Advancement
Relationship with peers	Growth

Factors Affecting Job Attitudes

Herzberg reasoned that because the factors causing satisfaction are different from those causing dissatisfaction, the two feelings cannot simply be treated as opposites of one another. The opposite of satisfaction is not dissatisfaction, but rather, no satisfaction. Similarly, the opposite of dissatisfaction is no dissatisfaction. There are physiological needs that can be fulfilled by money, for example, food and shelter. Second, there is the psychological need to achieve and grow, and this need is fulfilled by activities that cause one to grow. From the above table, one observes that the factors that determine dissatisfaction or no dissatisfaction are not part of the work itself, but rather, are external factors. Herzberg often referred to these hygiene factors as *KITA* factors, where KITA is an acronym for *kick in the a…* , the process of providing incentives or a threat of punishment to cause someone to do something. Herzberg argues that these provide only short-run success because the motivating factors that determine satisfaction or no satisfaction are intrinsic to the job itself and do not result from carrot and stick incentives.

Implications for Management

If the motivation-hygiene theory holds, management not only must provide hygiene factors to avoid employee dissatisfaction, but also must provide factors intrinsic to the work itself for employees to be satisfied with their jobs. Herzberg argued that job enrichment is required for intrinsic motivation and that it is a continuous management process. According to Herzberg:

- The job should have sufficient challenge to utilize the full ability of the employee.
- Employees who demonstrate increasing levels of ability should be given increasing levels of responsibility.
- If a job cannot be designed to use an employee's full abilities, then the firm should consider automating the task or replacing the employee with one who has a lower level of skill. If a person cannot be fully utilized, then there will be a motivation problem.

Critics of Herzberg's theory argue that the two-factor result is observed because it is natural for people to take credit for satisfaction and to blame dissatisfaction on external factors. Furthermore, job satisfaction does not necessarily imply a high level of motivation or productivity.

As part of the motivational process, it is extremely important to provide feedback and guidance at regular intervals. Regular feedback eliminates the process of blindsiding, where an employee thinks they are doing a good job only to find out at evaluation time that their performance is substandard. Known expectations are an important part of motivation, so the employee is not set up for failure.

The company mission and vision should be in alignment with expectations. Most importantly, positive feedback and reward should be employed.

TIME MANAGEMENT

Many publications on time management are available. However, this is one of the most important skills one can have as a new manager. Most of the time, tasks and assignments the manager has go beyond the time available for them.

One of the biggest interruptions is drop-in visitors. You will also spend much unplanned time putting out fires. Although it may be difficult, it is important to try to stick to your priorities. Also, when possible, do not take on the work of others.

Orientation by your immediate supervisor is a good idea. Find out what his or her priorities are. Try to establish documented expectations, goals, job description, and other factors, and ask for periodic evaluation and feedback from your boss.

IMAGINATION

Imagination in management is an often overlooked but very important factor. It can come into play in many facets of management—problem solutions, marketing, conflict resolution, and so on (see Graphic 2.1). Thinking out of the box should be

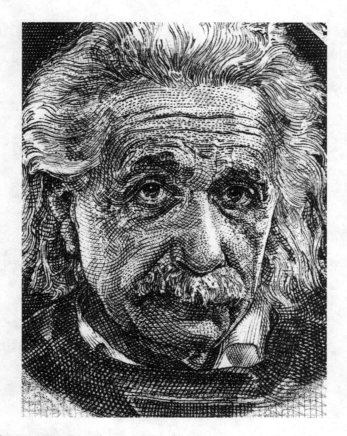

GRAPHIC 2.1 Albert Einstein valued "imagination over knowledge."

encouraged when appropriate. It is a known fact that Albert Einstein valued imagination over knowledge.

REFERENCES

1. Dawn Oetjen. Conflict Management. doetjen@mail.ucf.edu
2. *Ibid.*
3. Susan M. Heathfield. Delegation as a Leadership Style: Tips for Effective Delegation. About.com http://humanresources.about.com/cs/manageperformance/a/delegation.htm

3 Stress Management and Working with Radiologists

STRESS MANAGEMENT

An important skill to master for the new manager is *stress management*. There are many sources of management stress. This includes former peers, who, as discussed previously, may have a variety of issues with the new manager. A variety of stressors come from another source: the new boss, who will expect communication and reporting, and will put demands on the new manager, such as deadlines and projects. These will be constantly shifting in most cases. In addition, the new manager now has a new peer group, with whom to communicate, plan, and work beside. The level of day-to-day responsibility is greatly increased from the staff-level position the manager previously occupied.

The message to corporations: It is not only the "humane" thing to do to help workers manage stress, but it is also fiscally wise to provide outlets for excess stress on the job. Lack of any attempt at stress management could be costly and legally complicated (Graphic 3.1).

Recent studies have shown that workplace job morale is at its lowest. Approximately 60% of those surveyed feel that morale is not good. Emotional contagion research shows that people can catch bad moods from others. In addition, new research has found that there is a definite link between a sense of lack of control (no control over deadlines on multiple tasks) and increased heart attack risk. There is actually a sixfold increased heart attack risk due job deadline stress. Lack of reciprocal loyalty on corporation's part in honoring employee loyalty has resulted in greatly lowered morale.

Some stress facts are as follows:

- Stress is a major trigger to drinking and drug abuse (Graphic 3.2).[1]
- Twenty percent of people with heart disease also have depression.[2]
- Stress exacerbates gastrointestinal disorders.
- One out of four visits to the doctor's office deals with a physical illness that started off with stress.

HEALTH BENEFITS

Some benefits of managing stress properly are as follows:

- Turn back the biological clock by managing stress: relaxation slows aging.
- Attitude can influence survival time for people with terminal illnesses.
- Using a *relaxation response* improves mental performance (Graphic 3.3). Even aviation geniuses the Wright brothers took the day off before their historic flight.

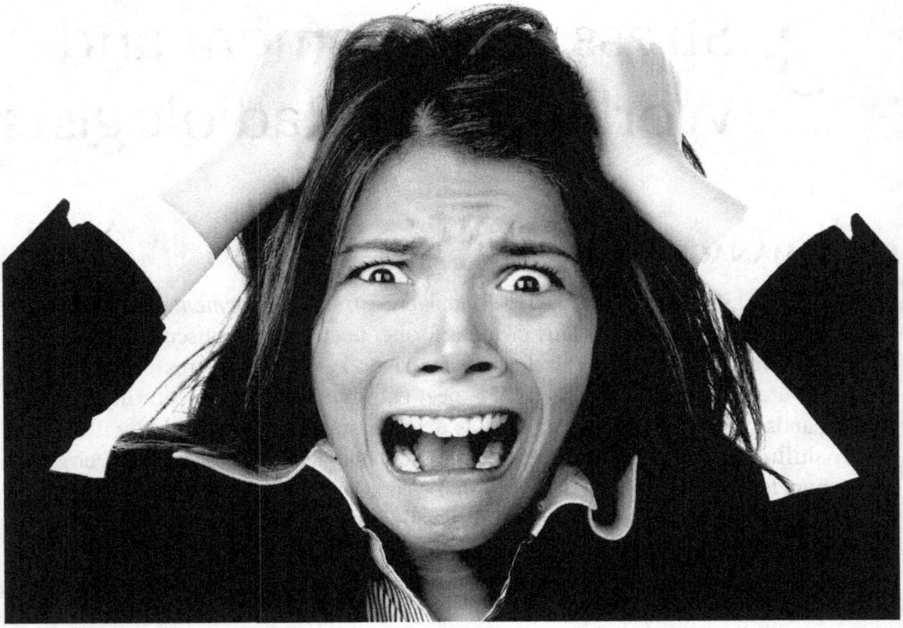

GRAPHIC 3.1 Stress can influence decisions.

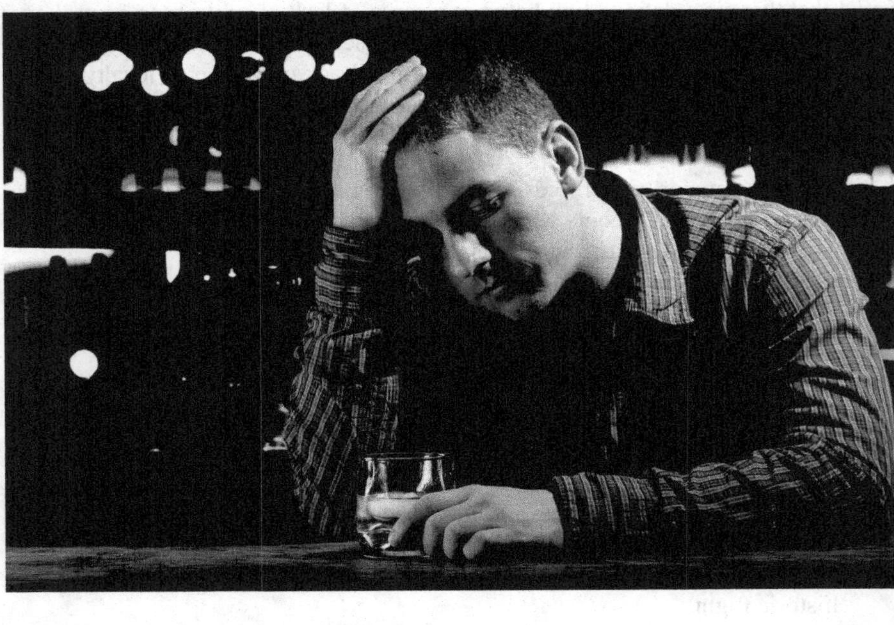

GRAPHIC 3.2 Stress can lead to bad habits.

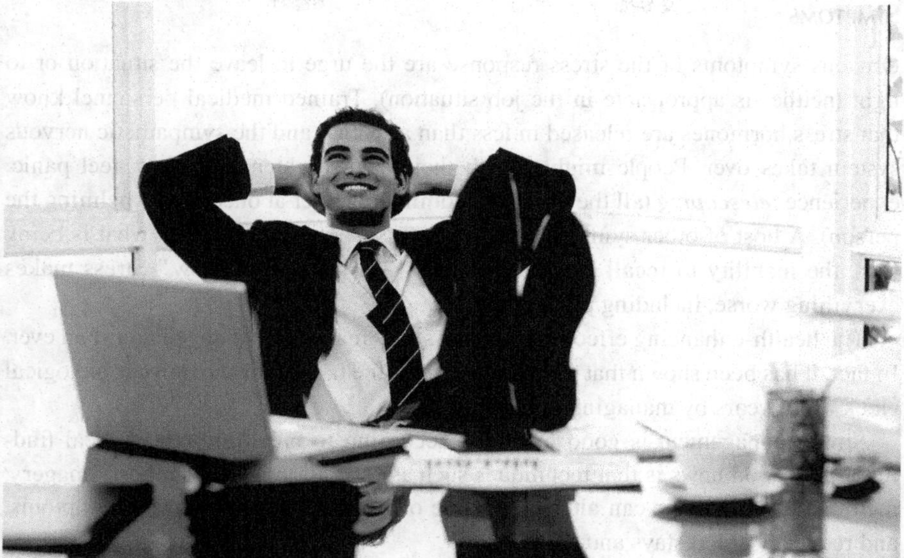

GRAPHIC 3.3 Stress managed properly.

Financial Benefits

Other benefits of managing stress are financial: avoiding stress-related lawsuits. For example, $50,000 was awarded by a state commissioner for "ongoing total disability compensations."[3]

Human Relations Benefits

Agreeable, stable employees are more successful and employable.[4]

New Development: Excess Stress Predicts Substance Abuse

Duke University Research[5] has revealed that stress is a major trigger to alcohol and substance abuse. To have a healthier workforce, reducing stress at work can even improve health habits at home. The reason stress increases the use of alcohol is that alcohol works within five minutes to calm down the burnt-out sympathetic nervous system's *fight or flight* response. Since it is obvious one cannot fight or run away at work, stress builds up, and alcohol provides immediate but unhealthy relief. It is obvious that workers who are recovering from stress-relief drinking cannot be at their peak. And excess job stress is partly to blame.

Symptoms

Obvious symptoms of the stress response are the urge to leave the situation or to fight (neither is appropriate in the job situation). Trained medical personnel know that stress hormones are released in less than a second and the sympathetic nervous system takes over. People might clench their teeth, tighten their fists, feel panic, experience *telescoping* (all the problems coming together at once, overwhelming the person). A host of other symptoms can appear, such as inattention to what is being said, the inability to recall information that "you know you know." Stress makes everything worse, including physical health.

The health-enhancing effects of positive stress management are clearer than ever. In fact, it has been shown that you can turn back the hands of time on your biological clock by 16 years by managing stress.[6]

Stress management is good medicine according to breakthrough medical findings.[7] The good news is that techniques such as relaxation, group support, imagery, meditation, and prayer can alter the course of some illnesses, decrease symptoms, and reduce hospital stays and medication.

Stress management makes you smarter, according to Dr. Herbert Benson.[8] Using the *relaxation response*, developed by Herbert Benson, M.D., at Harvard Medical School, improves mental performance. Basically, the relaxation response involves concentrating on one single thought for 20 minutes. The Harvard mantra is the word *one*. That is, just concentrating on the word *one* could be used as a focal thought for the relaxation response. This is in the 25th anniversary (2001) of Benson's book *The Relaxation Response*, which has sold four million copies.[9] His work on the relaxation response has revolutionized our understanding of the mind–body relationship.

Even aviation geniuses Orville and Wilbur Wright took the day off to relax before making their world-changing, first powered-airplane flight (Graphic 3.4).[10] Bestselling author Norman Vincent Peale advised, "Keep relaxed. The relaxed person is powerful."[11]

Research has shown that calmer brain-wave patterns are related to better mental functioning.[12] Agreeable, stable employees are more successful and employable.[13] As a shining example, NASA's astronaut motto is "Be overprepared and undertaxed," or understressed (Graphic 3.5).

Finally, unmanaged stress can hit a company where it hurts the most, in the pocketbook. Even if corporations don't address the humanitarian reasons to reduce debilitating stress in workers, insurance commissions can provide incentives to corporations to help workers manage stress. Workers have successfully won major cases (for example, $50,000) against companies that ignored pleas from workers that stress was affecting their physical health. It would seem fiscally prudent to have some type of organized stress management system in place in the event that a worker claims "stress is an occupational disease."

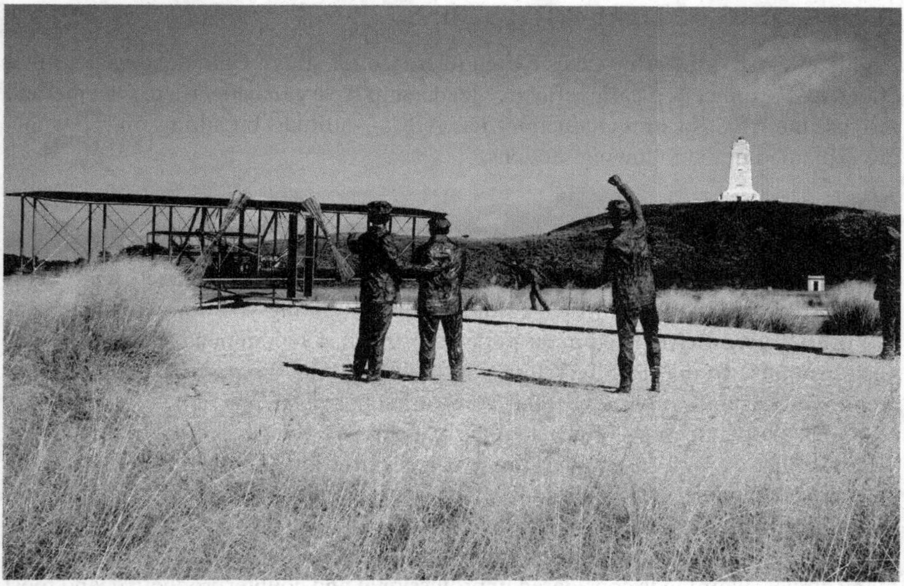

GRAPHIC 3.4 Wright Brothers monument.

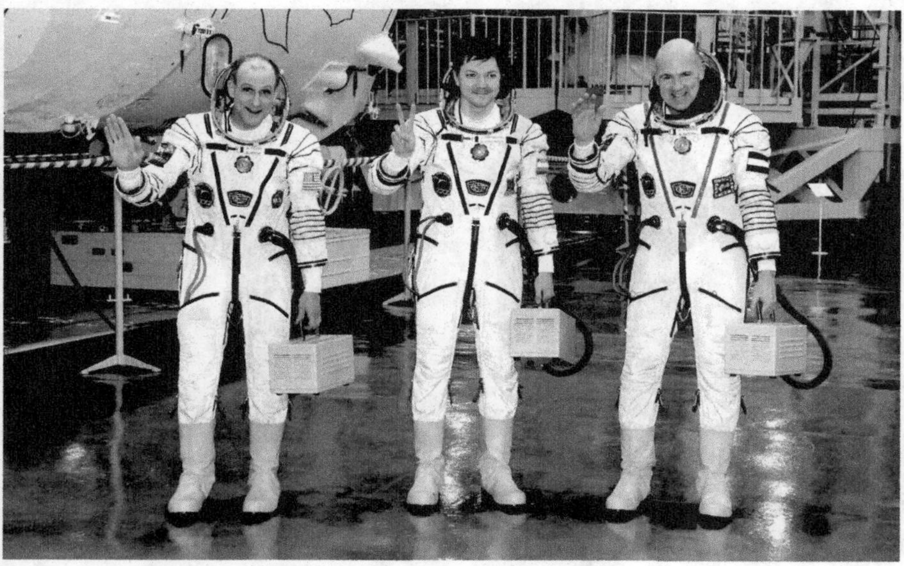

GRAPHIC 3.5 Astronauts know how to deal with stress.

TECHNIQUES TO DEAL WITH STRESS

Highly effective leadership takes a high tolerance for stress. Calm leaders are more effective. Fortunately, a calm, effective leadership style can be learned. One method is to use the ABCs of stress reduction. The ABCs—attitude, breathing, and choice—are explained in the following sections.

ATTITUDE

"Believe in yourself," advised Norman Vincent Peale.[14] Say to yourself with confidence, "I know I can!" Your own attitude is the only thing you have complete control over. To see if you need an attitude adjustment, I recommend the "Get Tough Test," available from Mentally Tough Corporate Training Programs.[15] If you have an employee assistance program available at work, take advantage of it.

Avoid "staff infections" by watching the company you keep. That is, a whining staff member can infect you with his or her negative attitudes within minutes. The best antidote against staff infections is to seek the company of positive and humorous people (Graphic 3.6).

Everyone needs a little time to "unwhine" or vent, but use common sense. In many circles, whining is considered unprofessional and counterproductive, and most people consider whining to be boring and annoying.

Convert bad stress into good stress just by thinking about it differently. Instead of saying, "I feel so stressed out," say, "I am so excited about the chance to … " Visualize perfection, such as your perfect vacation or a sweet victory. Athletes commonly consider the feeling of butterflies in the stomach to be an indication of

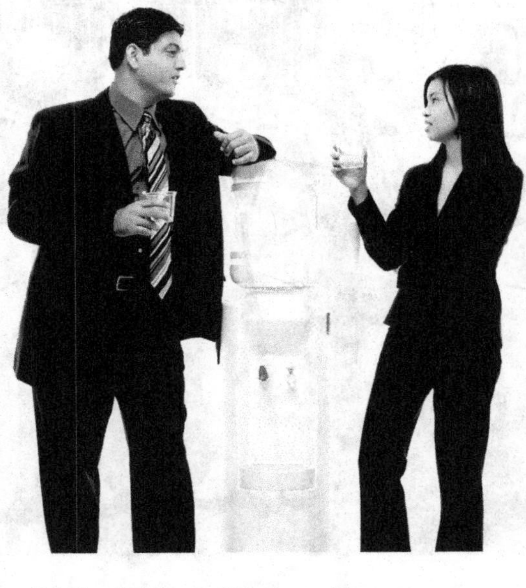

GRAPHIC 3.6 Possible "staff infection" in the making.

excitement and anticipation, not stress. Concentrate on improving your personal best, and don't worry about the rest. Get guidance if you need it.

Finally, remember that a single job activity is rarely life or death. You are judged generally on patterns of behavior and your ability to deal honestly with problems.

Breathing

The best cure for stress is right under your nose: breathing. If the Lamaze technique helps ease the pain of childbirth, deep breathing will help you at work (unless your job is worse than childbirth). Lamaze became popular in 1972.

Dr. Jon Kabat-Zinn,[16] director of a nationally acclaimed stress reduction program, has trained thousands to calm themselves under traumatically stressful conditions. The key to his method is to focus on the gentle rising and falling of your breathing. Insurance companies reimburse for this "breathing training" because of the highly successful results in reducing stress.

To calm down, just slow breathing using the number sequence 2-4-6.

Breathe in through the nose to the count of two (one-thousand one, one-thousand two); breathe out through the mouth to the count of four (one-thousand one, one-thousand two, one-thousand three, one-thousand four). Then repeat this sequence for a total of six times. That is, breathe in through the nose to the count of two, breathe out to the count of four, and do this six times.

Choice

Choose to control your work, not people (Graphic 3.7). Lack of control is the number one source of job stress. Not surprisingly, good time management is a key to job success, and job success reduces stress. Concentrate your efforts on job tasks and skills that will yield a high return on investment (ROI). Master soft skills (appearance, human relations, corporate culture), because practicing these skills can boost your personal job performance by 30 to 40% according to C. J. Taylor, president of The Mirror Ltd.[17]

Highly effective leadership takes a high tolerance for stress. Calm leaders are more effective. A calm, effective leadership style can be learned. The government bet on this fact with millions of taxpayer dollars funding the National/State Leadership Project in the 1980s. These future national leaders were taught to have a spirit of calm "unwarranted optimism" when facing problems.[18]

Know yourself: Are you possibly causing your own stress? Take the Effective Job-Stress Management Habits Checklist to see how much stress you are adding to the mix.

EFFECTIVE JOB-STRESS MANAGEMENT HABITS CHECKLIST

Do you consistently:

- Foster a "we attitude" rather than a "me attitude" [Yes] [No]
- Know what your supervisor wants [Yes] [No]

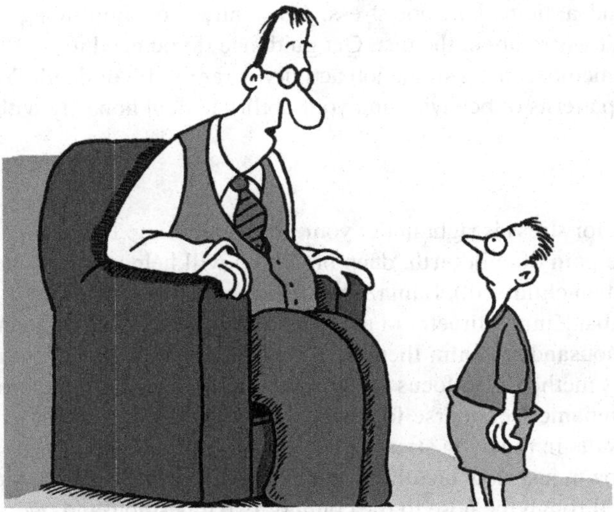
AS A DECISION MAKER, YOU'VE GOT TO WORK 24 HOURS A DAY. IT TAKES 10 MINUTES TO MAKE A DECISION AND 23 HOURS AND 50 MINUTES TO ASK YOURSELF IF YOU WERE RIGHT.

GRAPHIC 3.7

- Encourage communication/trust [Yes] [No]
- Practice clutter management [Yes] [No]
- Employ consistent (daily, weekly) time management [Yes] [No]
- Walk at break/take legitimate breaks [Yes] [No]
- Use a relaxation technique [Yes] [No]
- Deal with difficult people/conflict effectively [Yes] [No]
- Use problem solving and conflict resolution [Yes] [No]
- Engage in continual professional development [Yes] [No]

A Yes score of 9–10 = Model employee. A Yes score of 7–8 = Keep up the good work. A Yes score of 5–6 = Need improvement. A Yes score of 4 or less = Reexamine your priorities. [19]

Since lack of control over a work situation is the number one cause of job stress, perhaps taking a self-examination would be helpful to see how much control you do have. If you are trying the 10 job-stress management tips above and you are hitting a brick wall, you may be dealing with a modern Niccolo Machiavelli,[20] who doesn't respond to normal human emotions. Then it is time to contact your employee assistance program and start looking for a new job.

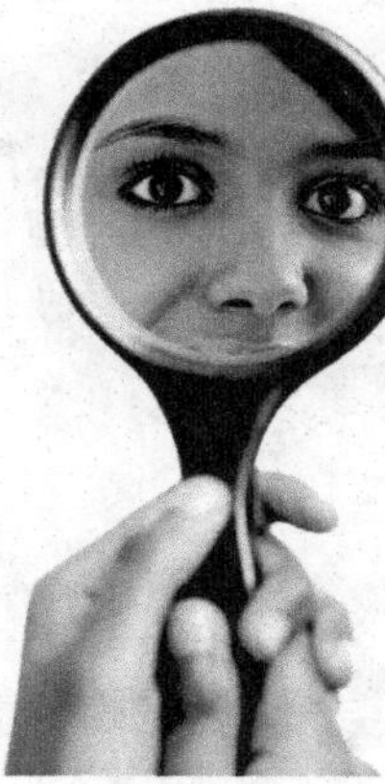

GRAPHIC 3.8 Examine your communication style.

For a true "x-ray" of your leadership strengths and needs on the job, contact the Center for Creative Leadership in Greensboro, North Carolina.* This organization is fine-tuned to develop the best leaders by pinpointing strengths and needs through a very thorough procedure. Good leadership is so essential that the Center for Creative Leadership claims that great leadership can increase employee retention by 73% and can affect the bottom line by 66%. Again, this type of in-depth analysis will help you understand if a possible source of job stress is *you* (Graphic 3.8).

WORKING WITH RADIOLOGISTS

The new manager will soon discover a different perspective and relationship with radiologists than they had when working as a technologist (Graphic 3.9). It is important to understand the relationship from the radiologist's perspective. Radiologists are under very high stress levels. Typically, they have limited training in areas outside the clinical realm. In addition, they are very highly specialized in clinical areas. Radiologists are patient centered, and managers must be business centered. High manager visibility in the department is important to radiologists.

The most important skill to be utilized when dealing with radiologists is communication.

Radiologists, just like everyone else, have different personalities. Learning these personalities and how to deal with each individual can contribute greatly to a manager's effectiveness. When discussing issues with radiologists, utilize what, when, where, and the priority of each issue or concern. Use common denominators in language that they can understand. When discussing coding, billing, and other related issues that are businesslike in nature, avoid jargon. Typically, radiologist input is vital when considering large capital purchases. Employ honest, straightforward communication when dealing with capital purchases. For example, make sure all of the

* (1 Leadership Pl., Greensboro, NC 27410; phone 336-545-2810; http://www.ccl.org/leadership/index.aspx).

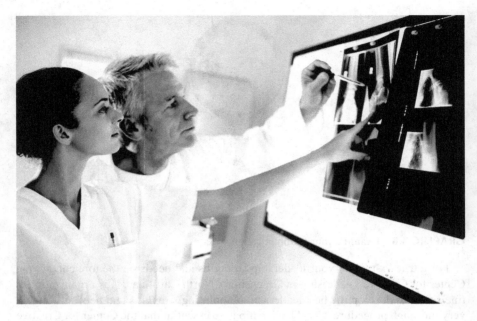

GRAPHIC 3.9 Radiologists are highly specialized in clinical areas.

weaknesses of the equipment are made known to them. This helps them to give the best input, and also avoids issues later when a problem or design weakness is discovered, especially right in the midst of a procedure!

When discussing issues, try to have all the facts and suggested solutions. Solution suggestions can be solicited from staff in many cases.

Some understanding of the radiologist's practice is helpful. These include clinical concerns, financial concerns, outpatient facility and joint venture concerns, and others.

Radiologists many times will have a financial interest in various entities, so it is important to keep them informed and to understand what their concerns are.

One often overlooked but extremely important fact is intrapractice cultural concerns. Differing personalities and interests, and especially the perception of fairness for issues such as pay, scheduling assignments, and time off need to be understood to an extent by the manager. In the past, it was typical for new radiologists in a practice to be financially oriented, taking extra calls, and so forth to help them buy their way into the group and establish equity. In recent times, lifestyle has become much more important. They now value time off to be with their families much more than financial gain.

Staff and administration interactions with radiologists will differ from those of the manager. It is important to understand the radiologist's perspective on these interactions. This will include financial, logistical, and clinical concerns.

REFERENCES

1. Dr. Paul Nagy, 2010, Duke University.
2. Harvard Medical School. 2003. Can a troubled mind spell trouble for the heart? *Harvard Mental Health Letter*. 19:10 (April), 1-3.
3. Paragraph 3, Page 12, I.C. 018642, filed May 20, 2002.
4. McDaniel, M. A., & Frei, R. 1994. *The validity of customer service orientation measures in employee selection: A comprehensive review and meta-analysis*. Paper presented at the Ninth Annual Conference of the Society of Industrial and Organizational Psychology, Inc., Nashville, TN, April.
5. Nagy, 2010.
6. Roizen, M. F. RealAge Benefits. Accessed on the Internet on Feb. 28, 2003 (http://www.realage.com/). and Roizen, M. F. 1999. Real Age: Are you as young as you càn be? New York, NY: Harper Collins.
7. Cousins, N. 1989. Head first—The biology of hope. New York: E.P. Dutton. Marucha, P. T., Kiecolt-Glaser, J. K.,& Favagehi, M. 1998. Mucosal wound healing is impaired by examination stress. *Psychosomatic Medicine* 60, 362–365.
8. Benson, H., Kornhaber, A., Kornhaber, C., Le Chanu, M., Zuttermeister, P. C., Myers, P., & Friedman, R. 1994. Increases in positive psychological characteristics with a new relaxation response curriculum in high school students. 1994. The *Journal of Research and Development in Education* 27:4, 226–231.
9. Benson, H., and Klipper, M. 1976. *The relaxation response*. New York: Avon Books.
10. Moolman, V. 1980. *The epic of flight. The road to Kitty Hawk*. Alexandria, VA: Time-Life Books. P. 150.
11. Peale, N.V. 1975.Ten steps to success: Positive thinking for a time like this. How to have what it takes. (2003, April), Carmel, NY: Positive Thinking. P. 22.
12. Haier, 2006; optimists live 7.5 years longer.
13. McDaniel, M. A., & Frei, R. 1994. *The validity of customer service orientation measures in employee selection: A comprehensive review and meta-analysis*. Paper presented at the Ninth Annual Conference of the Society of Industrial and Organizational Psychology, Inc., Nashville, TN, April.
14. Peale, 1992.
15. LGE Performance Systems, Inc. 2002. Get Tough Test. 9757 Lake Nona Road, Orlando, FL 32827, 407/438-9911; 800/LGE-PROG.
16. Kabat-Zinn, J. 1990. *Full catastrophe living: Using the wisdom of your body and mind to face stress, pain, and illness*. New York: Random House/Bantam Dell.
17. Taylor, C. J. 2003, March. *The "softest" skills for trainers that impact the bottom line*. Greensboro, NC: American Society for Training and Development.
18. Tannenbaum, A. J. 1983. *Gifted children: Psychological and educational perspectives*. New York: Macmillan. P. 37.
19. Rubenzer, R. L. 2003. *How the best handle stress*. Cornelius, NC: Warren Publishing. Pp. 52–53.
20. Bing, 2000.

Section II

Human Resource Management

4 Recruiting, Interviewing, and Hiring

Over the past decades shortages have occurred in almost all disciplines in medical imaging. Conversely, so have overages. These occur because of change in demand, which can be caused by several factors including changes in technology, aging population, number of programs producing graduates of imaging disciplines, the economy in general, and increase in utilization (computed tomography or CT, magnetic resonance imaging or MRI). It has been stated that the demand for imaging services will be increasing greatly in the future due to the ramifications of "Obamacare," (Patient Protection and Affordable Care Act of 2010) which will include a much higher percentage of the population having access to care.

Lower staffing ratios have been the rule due to increased pressures on reducing cost. The American Healthcare Radiology Administrators (AHRA) publishes staffing benchmarks and ratios by modality every few years. These statistics typically are broken down by different sizes of institutions, areas of the country, and a variety of other factors. These survey results are a good place for the manager to start in assessing staffing levels. However, situations that are unique to each institution will ultimately decide the correct staffing levels.

When a position is to be filled, some work should be complete before the process begins. This includes development and sign-off on the following:

- Job description
- Pay and benefits level
- Orientation checklist
- Institution and department mission, vision, and values statements
- Interview schedule and participants
- Organizational chart

To properly ascertain the job requirements, a job analysis should be performed. See Sample Job Analyis in box below.

SAMPLE JOB ANALYSIS FORM[1]

PURPOSE AND INSTRUCTIONS

The purpose of the study is to obtain current information on your job based on a review of job duties and responsibilities. An important concept of a job analysis is that the analysis is conducted of the job, not the person.

Because you know your duties and responsibilities better than anyone else, we need your help to get an accurate description of your job. We are asking you to complete this questionnaire about your job duties. The questionnaire does not ask about your job performance; but only what your job requires you to do.

Please complete this questionnaire as honestly, completely, and accurately as you can. Base your answers on what is normal to your current job, not special projects or temporary assignment duties, unless these tasks are a regular part of your job. If two answers seem to fit your situation, select the one that works best. When answering the questions, imagine you are describing your job to a neighbor, friend, or someone just hired for your position.

Job title: ____________

Department: ____________

How long have you been in your current position?: ____years ____ months

Reports to: ____________

GENERAL PURPOSE OF THE JOB

(Briefly describe the job's primary purpose or contribution to the department or the organization.)

ESSENTIAL DUTIES AND RESPONSIBILITIES

Describe specific job responsibilities and duties, listing the most important first. Use a separate statement for each responsibility. Most positions can be described in 8–10 major responsibility areas. Combine minor or occasional duties in one last statement. Give a best estimate of average percentage of time each responsibility takes; however, do not include a duty that occupies 5 percent or less of your time unless it is an essential part of the job. Each statement should be brief and concise, beginning with an action verb. Tables 4.1 and 4.2 show two different examples.

SUPERVISORY RESPONSIBILITIES

Does this job have supervisory responsibilities? ____ Yes ____ No

How many employees, in total, report to this job? ____

Are there subordinate supervisors reporting to this job? ____ Yes _ No

If yes, how many subordinate supervisors report to this job? ____

TABLE 4.1
Job Analysis 1

— Example Job Analysis —	Percent (%) of Time
Secretary	
1. Performs a variety of typing duties including standard letters, reports, and forms.	25%
2. Takes and transcribes dictation. Composes letters and memos as directed.	25%
3. Maintains departmental files; ensures that all records are updated and modified as necessary.	20%
4. Answers the telephone and greets visitors.	20%
5. Makes travel arrangements.	10%
	100%

Source: Patricia Dougherty of the Weston Group. With permission.

TABLE 4.2
Job Analysis 2

List Most Important Duties First	Percent (%) of Time
Transporting and assisting in moving patients for MRI and CT. Delivers patient care based upon current, comprehensive, professional knowledge skills.	
Identifies patients using double identifiers for patient safety. Able to prepare the imaging rooms—cleaning and stocking.	
Assists the technologists in performing a variety of technical procedures including preparation of equipment according to procedure. Able to assist patients—ambulation and transfers.	
Provides direct patient care under the supervision and coordination with technologist for the correct prep and setup of the imaging rooms.	
Assists in setup for interventional procedures throughout the imaging department, as requested. Assists radiology nurse and/or technologists in care of patients during interventional procedures. Sets up sterile trays and assists the radiologist during invasive procedures.	
Stocks and cleans rooms in CT, MRI, and X-ray.	
Ordering and stocking supplies for CT, MRI, and X-ray.	
Other job duties—confirms patients for CT and MRI when scheduler is off in the HIS scheduling module. Able to verify the patient order is correct.	
Helps with Nighthawk reports and checks that reports are read and in the system.	
Identifies patients using double identifiers for patient safety.	
Total	100%

Source: Patricia Dougherty of the Weston Group. With permission.

TABLE 4.3
Job Analysis 3

Name	Title	Purpose
	Radiology Supervisor	
	Lead CT Tech	Help process flow of patient care
	Lead MRI Tech	Help process flow of patients and MRI breast positioning

Source: Patricia Dougherty of the Weston Group. With permission.

FROM WHOM DO YOU NORMALLY RECEIVE WORK ASSIGNMENTS?

Refer to Table 4.3.

EDUCATION AND/OR EXPERIENCE

Select the level of education and/or experience needed to successfully accomplish the essential duties of this job.

__Level 1: No prior experience or training.
__Level 2: Less than high school education; or up to one month related experience or training; or equivalent combination of education and experience.
__Level 3: High school diploma or general education degree (GED); or one to three months' related experience and/or training; or equivalent combination of education and experience.
__Level 4: One-year certificate from college or technical school; or three to six months' related experience and/or training; or equivalent combination of education and experience.
__Level 5: Associate's degree (A.A.) or equivalent from two-year college or technical school; or six months' to one year related experience and/or training; or equivalent combination of education and experience.
__Level 6: Bachelor's degree (B.A.) from four-year college or university; or one to two years' related experience and/or training; or equivalent combination of education and experience.
__Level 7: This position requires ________ education and/or __ years of experience.

Language Skills

Select the level of language (ability to read, write, and speak) needed to successfully accomplish the essential duties of this job.

__Level 1: Ability to read a limited number of two- and three-syllable words and to recognize similarities and differences between words and between series of numbers. Ability to print and speak simple sentences.

__Level 2: Ability to read and comprehend simple instructions, short correspondence, and memos. Ability to write simple correspondence. Ability to effectively present information in one-on-one and small group situations to customers, clients, and other employees of the organization.

__Level 3: Ability to read and interpret documents such as safety rules, operating and maintenance instructions, and procedure manuals. Ability to write routine reports and correspondence. Ability to speak effectively before groups of customers or employees of organization.

__Level 4: Ability to read, analyze, and interpret general business periodicals, professional journals, technical procedures, or governmental regulations. Ability to write reports, business correspondence, and procedure manuals. Ability to effectively present information and respond to questions from groups of managers, clients, customers, and the general public.

Mathematical Skills

Select the level of mathematical skills and ability needed to successfully accomplish the essential duties of this job.

__Level 1, Minimum skills: Ability to add and subtract two digit numbers and to multiply and divide with 10s and 100s. Ability to perform these operations using units of American money and weight measurement, volume, and distance.

__Level 2, Basic skills: Ability to add, subtract, multiply, and divide in all units of measure, using whole numbers, common fractions, and decimals. Ability to compute rate, ratio, and percent and to draw and interpret bar graphs.

__Level 3, Intermediate skills: Ability to calculate figures and amounts such as discounts, interest, commissions, proportions, percentages, area, circumference, and volume. Ability to apply concepts of basic algebra and geometry.

__Level 4, High skills: Ability to work with mathematical concepts such as probability and statistical inference, and fundamentals of plane and solid geometry and trigonometry. Ability to apply concepts such as fractions, percentages, ratios, and proportions to practical situations.

Reasoning Ability

Select the level of reasoning skills and abilities needed to successfully accomplish the essential duties of this job.

__Level 1, Minimum skills: Ability to apply commonsense understanding to carry out simple one- or two-step instructions. Ability to deal with standardized situations with only occasional or no variables.

__Level 2, Basic skills: Ability to apply commonsense understanding to carry out detailed but uninvolved written or oral instructions. Ability to deal with problems involving a few concrete variables in standardized situations.

__Level 3, Intermediate skills: Ability to apply commonsense understanding to carry out instructions furnished in written, oral, or diagram form. Ability to deal with problems involving several concrete variables in standardized situations.

__Level 4, High skills: Ability to solve practical problems and deal with a variety of concrete variables in situations where only limited standardization exists. Ability to interpret a variety of instructions furnished in written, oral, diagram, or schedule form.

__Level 5, Very high skills: Ability to define problems, collect data, establish facts, and draw valid conclusions. Ability to interpret an extensive variety of technical instructions in mathematical or diagram form and deal with several abstract and concrete variables.

Certificates, Licenses, Registrations

List the licenses, certificates, and registrations that are required to perform the essential duties of this job. (Examples: commercial driver's license, boiler operator, food handler permit, etc. Refer to Table 4.4.)

Other Skills, Abilities or Qualifications

List other items not already previously mentioned. (Refer to Table 4.5.)

PHYSICAL DEMANDS

How much on-the-job time is spent on the following physical activities? Show the time by checking the appropriate boxes in Table 4.6.

TABLE 4.4
Job Analysis 4

CPR—works directly in patient care

CNA or EMT Basic State License preferred within 18 months of hiring

Source: Patricia Dougherty of the Weston Group. With permission.

TABLE 4.5
Job Analysis 5

Helpful to have computer knowledge of Excel and Word; ability to write, read, and comprehend simple instructions and memos. Excellent patient care skills. Able to communicate with patients, family members, caregivers, and physicians.

One year experience in healthcare is preferred, ability to lift/transfer patient, frequently requires rotating torso in all directions. Able to learn sterile techniques to set up trays for biopsies.

Preferred to have knowledge of medical terminology, ability to apply common sense to carry out instructions. Ability to speak and hear in normal range.

Source: Patricia Dougherty of the Weston Group. With permission.

TABLE 4.6
Job Analysis 6

	On-the-Job Time (Per Workday)				
Condition	**None**	**Under 1/3**	**1/3**	**To 2/3**	**Over 2/3**
Stand					
Walk					
Sit					
Use hands to finger, handle, or feel					
Reach with hands and arms					
Climb or balance					
Stoop, kneel, crouch, or crawl					
Talk or hear					
Taste or smell					

Source: Patricia Dougherty of the Weston Group. With permission.

Does this job require that weight be lifted or force be exerted? If so, how much and how often? Check the appropriate boxes in Table 4.7.

Please give examples of items that must be lifted (refer to Table 4.8).

Does this job have any special vision requirements? Check all that apply:

__ Close vision (clear vision at 20 inches or less)
__ Distance vision (clear vision at 20 feet or more)
__ Color vision (ability to identify and distinguish colors)
__ Peripheral vision (ability to observe an area that can be seen up and down or to the left and right while eyes are fixed on a given point)
__ Depth perception (three-dimensional vision, ability to judge distances and spatial relationships)

TABLE 4.7
Job Analysis 7

Condition	None	Under 1/3	1/3	To 2/3	Over 2/3
	On-the-Job Time (Per Workday)				
Must be able to lift or move weights:					
Up to 10 pounds					
Up to 25 pounds					
Up to 50 pounds					
Up to 100 pounds					
More than 100 pounds					

Source: Patricia Dougherty of the Weston Group. With permission.

TABLE 4.8
Job Analysis 8

Transferring patients to and from wheelchairs and stretchers onto tables—full lifting, bending, pushing, and pulling.
Stocking the room for drinking contrast, films, and supplies. Reaching to put supplies away.

Source: Patricia Dougherty of the Weston Group. With permission.

__ Ability to adjust focus (ability to adjust the eye to bring an object into sharp focus)
__ No special vision requirements

Make notes on the specific job duties that require the physical demands selected above.

WORK ENVIRONMENT

How much exposure to environmental conditions does this job require? Show the amount of on-the-job time by checking the appropriate boxes in Table 4.9.

How much noise is typical for the work environment of this job? Check the appropriate level below:

__ Very quiet conditions (examples: forest trail, isolation booth for hearing test)
__ Quiet conditions (examples: library, private office)
__ Moderate noise (examples: business office with computers and printers, light traffic)

TABLE 4.9
Job Analysis 9

Condition	None	Under 1/3	1/3	To 2/3	Over 2/3
	On-the-Job Time (Per Workday)				
Wet or humid conditions (nonweather)					
Work near moving mechanical parts					
Work in high, precarious places					
Fumes or airborne particles					
Toxic or caustic chemicals					
Outdoor weather conditions					
Extreme cold (nonweather)					
Extreme heat (nonweather)					
Risk of electrical shock					
Work with explosives					
Risk of radiation					
Vibration					

Source: Patricia Dougherty of the Weston Group. With permission.

— Loud noise (examples: metal can manufacturing department, large earth-moving equipment, jackhammer work, front row at rock concert)

ADDITIONAL INFORMATION

Include any other information that will aid in the preparation of an accurate description of this job.

Ability to problem solve when patient complaints arise
Ability to work by self and with others
Able to communicate with patients, caregivers, and physicians
Able to look at process flow and make suggestions to improve work flows
Assess strengths and weaknesses—willing to pursue additional training and opportunity for developing and improving
Accept feedback from others with a positive attitude
Able to make sound judgments and able to support and handle situations as they arise
Motivated—willing to help out in all of imaging department
Diversity—respectful and sensitive to cultural diversity
Self-motivated

Form Prepared By:
Name ______________________ Title ______________________ Date ________
Form Reviewed By:
Name ______________________ Title ______________________ Date ________

Alternatively, job descriptions can be obtained from peers and modified to fit the institution's particular needs and requirements.

JOB DESCRIPTION

The job description needs to contain the mission, vision, and values of the hiring organization (these are described in Chapter 13).

The next section should be a summary, which explains in a paragraph what the job entails.

The third section should describe who the caregiver supervises, if any, who the caregiver is responsible to, and whom the caregiver is evaluated by.

The fourth section describes the professional qualifications of the job, such as training and licensure.

The fifth section describes personal attributes, such as being a fast learner and being able to think on one's feet (see sample job description).

The next section describes the physical requirements, such as bending and lifting. This section serves several purposes. First, it describes the physical attributes necessary to perform the job. This can alert a candidate to the possibility that he or she may not be able to perform all of the required tasks. In addition, it acts as a preventive measure so the caregiver can know what to expect and be prepared for it.

The document should also contain information as to the expected working hours and shifts, as much as can reasonably be stated generically.

A "Special Considerations" area should be included. It is a catchall that documents further expectations. For an idea of what this should contain, please see the sample job description below.

Performance standards should be described. This will lay out the performance expectations. These are also mirrored in the periodic evaluation document.

Lastly, the document should be reviewed and signed off by the department director, medical director, and human resources department.

It is now a Joint Commission requirement that all imaging job descriptions be reviewed and signed off at a general medical executive staff meeting. These signoffs can also be part of the job description.

A sample job description for a staff radiologic technologist follows in box, below.

REGIONAL MEDICAL CENTER

JOB DESCRIPTION

Radiology Tech I (Radiographer)

Mission:
Vision:
Values:

JOB SUMMARY

Administers procedures and diagnostic evaluations of patients requiring radiographic services. Utilizes the hospital information system (HIS) and other office equipment. Follows hospital and departmental policies and procedures regarding patient information documentation, confidentiality, and patient assessment, including communication of pain management needs. Maintains professional ethics standards, demonstrates professional attitude and behavior, and complies with corporate compliance requirements. Participates in performance improvement activities within the hospital and department and observes all safety and infection control practices. Meets customer service criteria. Category I BBP (blood-borne pathogens) and radiation exposure is probable with patient or patient specimen interaction.

JOB RELATIONSHIP

1. Supervises: students
2. Responsible to: radiology department director, radiology supervisor
3. Evaluated by: radiology department director, radiology supervisor

QUALIFICATIONS

1. Professional:
   a. Current national certification in radiography by the American Registry of Radiologic Technologists (ARRT).
   b. Current state license.
   c. Appropriate experience of one year desired but not essential.
   d. Willingness to work and/or cross-train in other modalities highly preferred.
   e. Current CPR certification—must be obtained within three months of employment.
2. Personal:
   a. Meets physical requirements to perform radiographic procedures and related tasks.
   b. Demonstrates ability to work under minimal supervision.
   c. Relates well with doctors and other hospital staff.

d. Is a quick aggressive learner and is proactive.
e. Is familiar with all radiographic procedures and equipment, enabling the technologist to perform any radiographic procedure.
f. Demonstrates ability to provide age-specific care during imaging procedures.

3. Physical: The physical demands described here are representative of those that must be met by the caregiver to successfully perform the essential functions of this job. Reasonable accommodations may be made to enable individuals with disabilities to perform the essential functions.
   a. Physical requirements:
      i. Standing/walking: performed routinely.
      ii. Sitting: frequently for periods less than 1 hour.
      iii. Lifting/carrying: frequently.
      iv. Torso rotation: frequently moves torso in all directions.
      v. Bending/stooping: frequently.
      vi. Squatting/crouching/kneeling: performed routinely.
      vii. Grasping/handling/fingering: performed routinely.
      viii. Communication: able to speak and hear within normal range.
      ix. Vision: frequent viewing of computer screens.
   b. Working conditions:
      i. Exposed to latex products routinely.
      ii. Potential exposure to blood-borne pathogens.
      iii. Climate controlled environment.
4. Work schedule:
   a. Job requires caregiver to work different shifts, days of weeks, holidays, call, and weekends, as assigned.
   b. Must be flexible with scheduling.

SPECIAL CONSIDERATIONS

1. The age legend below will apply to this position since the technologist will interact with a variety of patients during the course of the day.

Infant	0 months—1 year
Pediatric	13 months—12 years
Adolescent	13 years—17 years
Adult	18 years—64 years
Older Adult	65 years +

2. The caregiver performs within the prescribed limits of the hospital's/department's ethics and compliance program and is responsible to observe and report compliance variances to his/her immediate supervisor or upward through the chain of command, the compliance coordinator, or the hospital hotline.
3. The caregiver observes hospital safety and infection control policies.
4. The caregiver likely will be exposed to contact with patients or patient specimens, for example, blood, body fluids, or nonintact skin or tissue specimens on a routine basis. This type of exposure is considered a Category I BBP exposure.
5. The caregiver will be exposed to ionizing radiation in the course of job duties pertaining to interactions with patients or patient specimens.
6. The caregiver complies with the organizational values as follows:
   a. Compassion
   b. Customer focused
   c. Innovation
   d. Integrity
   e. Excellence
   f. Respect
7. The caregiver participates in hospital/department performance improvement activities.
8. The caregiver at all times maintains a positive attitude that is customer-service focused.
9. The caregiver participates in professional growth and development activities.

PERFORMANCE STANDARDS

1. Performs a variety of technical procedures that require independent judgment with ingenuity and initiative to apply prescribed exposure parameters for radiographic procedures according to patient age, mental, and physical status.
2. Maintains rooms and radiology department with adequate supplies and is responsible for an orderly working area.
3. Maintains adequate records as directed to ensure safety and proper care of patients and diagnostic quality of radiographs.
4. Performs callback duties when required and works assigned shifts as scheduled.
5. Assist physicians during procedures while maintaining a sterile field, when required.
6. Consistently uses radiation protection measures such as time, collimation, shielding, and distance.

7. Shows proof of continuing education as required by the state of ________ (where required) and the American Registry of Radiologic Technologists.
8. Passes the annual competency evaluations.
9. Maintains a safe environment for him-/herself, other caregivers, and patients.
10. Assesses patients' needs relevant to radiographic procedures.
11. Performs procedures with competence and ease to instill confidence in patients.
12. Maintains and records all pertinent information needed to complete the caregivers' job for all systems.
13. Follows hospital policy regarding pain management and the use of restraints for patients.
14. Demonstrates working knowledge of the HIS and picture archiving and communication system (PACS).
15. Performs all other tasks as assigned by the radiography section head, radiology supervisor, and/or radiology department director.

I understand that I will be required to become proficient and competent in radiology policies and procedures.

I have received and read a copy of my job descriptions and the correlating evaluation criteria and agree to abide by the contents.

________________________ ____

Date Signature

____

Printed Name

Director, Imaging Services

________________________ Medical Director, Radiology and Nuclear Medicine

RECRUITING

Recruiting effort will change with the times. Shortages and overages of available types of technologists will change over time. In almost all modalities, there is a cyclical nature to shortages and overages. These can vary in time depending on economic, legal, and other environmental changes.

As an example, in 2012 there was an overage of x-ray technologists. However, the number of schools offering certificates is steadily increasing. There are two-year certificate programs and four-year university-based bachelor programs. Schools advertise increasing demand due to aging baby boomers, increased regulation, and other reasons. This attracts first- and second-career students. However, because of the present economic conditions, baby boomers' staying in their careers, and other factors, the number of openings is limited.

It is important to do an "environmental scan" when putting together a recruiting plan. In the 1990s, there was an explosion in outpatient imaging centers. Later, due to legislative and economic conditions, many investors began shying away from ownership in these centers. Outpatient imaging center ownership has also changed from an enterprise that may be owned by a group of physicians and/or investors to joint venture with hospitals. All of this has decreased the present demand for imaging technologists.

The challenge becomes attracting the best candidates. The best way to accomplish this is to *differentiate* your institution from others. A variety of methods can help to accomplish this.

The size and type of institution (large or small hospital, large or small free-standing imaging clinic, doctor's office, etc.) will depend on how it is presented. For example, a free-standing center typically does not have late hours or call, which is attractive to many candidates. A hospital may promote variety and *cross-training opportunities*. Location can also be used—the attractiveness and homey atmosphere of a small institution and the cultural opportunities of an institution in a large city are examples.

In addition many institutions will offer *educational assistance* and *teaching* opportunities. Hospitals typically may have an affiliation agreement with a local school that will send students for clinical experience.

Flexible scheduling is attractive because it offers caregivers the ability to vary hours according to their lifestyle.

Compensation and benefits should also be attractors. *Sign-on and moving bonuses* may be offered as incentives.

An institution with very *high-tech equipment* is attractive to some candidates, so this should be emphasized if it exists.

There are many *resources* available to advertise openings. Most of these are online and consist of generalized and specialized job boards. Other places to advertise are imaging specialty sites such as Aunt Minnie, ASRT (American Society of Radiologic Technologists), state society boards, trade journals, and local newspapers.

It is important to include location, a condensed position responsibilities statement, and salary range in ads. Such things as relocation allowance can also be posted.

INTERVIEWING

The interview process is the opportunity to assess various candidates for an open position. Although interview results are an inexact science, an interview is the best tool currently available to ascertain the fit for an open position.

It is important that the director, manager, or supervisor work in concert with the human resources department. Human resources personnel are experts in this area and should be consulted frequently.

To start the process an *interview form* should be developed. This is important because a standard set of questions can be used with all candidates. There are also many legal ramifications during the interview process. These will be discussed in Chapter 5.

If possible, obtain input during development of the interview form from caregivers doing the same job that will be interviewed. Some questions can be open ended, which require the candidate to expound on the answer. Others can be close ended, which require a simple answer such as yes/no. A mock interview should be held to ascertain the efficacy of the interview form questions.

Notes should be kept during the interview process.

Typically, a candidate can be asked to elaborate on their *strengths and weaknesses*. Be careful, as many candidates will have preplanned answers. The goal is to get the most honest feedback possible from the candidate.

It is a good idea to present the candidate with a *hypothetical situation* to assess their knowledge and behavior as they relate to a departmental or patient care situation. For example, a question such as this can be posited: "Mrs. Jones comes in with her young daughter for an ankle x-ray. Her daughter is crying hysterically. What do you do?"

Next ask the candidate what their *short- and long-range goals* are. This will give the interviewer clues as to the intention on the candidate. For example, if the candidate states something like "I'd like to cross-train into MRI in the next few years," this gives the interviewer a clue that this candidate is planning to stay a while.

Also important is to ask the candidate why they are thinking of leaving their present position. An indirect answer can sometimes point to a hidden problem, such as the inability to get along with co-workers or management.

The interviewer can also ask about any special accomplishments the candidate wishes to present.

After the interview, answers should be rated on a scale—such as 1 to 5, with 1 being the poorest answer and 5 being the best. Interview scoring is a way to utilize impartiality and rate candidates properly. Divide the candidate's total score into minimal, meets, or exceeds requirements. Any gaps in employment should also be clarified.

Don't forget to trust your instincts. The interview process is imperfect, and anything that adds to the decision is useful.

A variety of topics cannot be discussed during the interview:

1. Race
2. Color
3. Sex
4. Religion
5. National origin
6. Birthplace
7. Age
8. Disability
9. Marital/family status

Some of the legislative acts regarding hiring practices are discussed in Chapter 5.

HIRING

After a candidate has been chosen, background checks should be performed. In addition, credentials, such as ARRT or ARDMS (American Registry for Diagnostic Medical Sonography) registration should be verified. Education should be verified.

After these requirements are met, if the candidate is interested, benefits should be explained, a copy of the job description given, and an offer made.

If the offer is accepted, the candidate should be given a copy of the institutional and/or departmental mission, vision, and values; departmental organization chart and goals; orientation manual; and an orientation checklist.

REFERENCE

1. Courtesy of Patricia Dougherty SPHR (Senior Professional in Human Resources), The Weston Group LLC.

5 Orientation, Coaching and Counseling—Legal Aspects

It is important to start an employee off feeling familiar and welcomed. Having an *orientation checklist* helps to ensure that the new hire is properly familiarized with the job and associated expectations.

One of the best ways to accomplish orientation is to assign an orientation coach. This can be another employee in the same position, or a supervisor.

To begin with, the new employee should be given a *general orientation* that defines logistics and layout of the department and facility. This should be followed by a *modality checklist,* which defines equipment and supplies unique to each individual modality (CT, MRI, etc.).

This should be followed by the *department routine and technique manuals.*

It is important that the new hire be familiarized with both the *facility and departmental policies and procedures.* A checklist for these should be developed.

To help the new individual understand their place in the organization, they should be given an *organizational chart* for the department that describes the positions and names the people associated with them.

The manager or supervisor should review the orientation and associated checklists with the employee at the end of the orientation period. At that point the new employee should sign the checklist, attesting to the fact the material has been reviewed. After signature by the person doing the orientation, a copy should be given to the employee, and one retained in the employee's personnel file (see Chart 5.1).

COACHING AND COUNSELING

Coaching and *counseling* are somewhat interchangeable terms. *Coaching* utilizes regular, documented feedback. At the beginning of the coaching process it is important that expectations are known. Motivational techniques should be used to encourage the employee to reach for higher performance levels.

Counseling happens when there are performance problems. This should be performed as a step prior to formalized corrective action. Coaching is usually required in the *progressive discipline* process. Legal entities will look for this process and documentation for it before an employee is dismissed, unless the dismissal is a flagrant violation of policy. During the coaching process, the reiteration of goals and expectations should occur, and the results of lack of improvement should be explained. In all cases, documentation must occur. It is also vital to have the caregiver sign the associated forms used.

LEGAL ASPECTS

Employment laws to be aware of are listed below.

A. For 1–14 employees:
   1. Title VII of the Civil Rights Act of 1964 (for employment agencies and labor organizations). See Item C for employers with 15–19 employees.
      - Related to nondiscrimination by national origin, race, religion, etc.
   2. Consumer Credit Protection Act of 1968
      - Nondiscriminatory disclosure of actual costs of borrowing money in laymen's terms
   3. Employee Polygraph Protection Act of 1988
      - Describes lie detectors and other devices that cannot be used in hiring/firing, etc.
   4. Employee Retirement Income Security Act (ERISA) of 1974 (if company offers benefits)
      - Delineates minimum standards for voluntarily established pension plans
   5. Equal Pay Act of 1963
      - Equal pay for equal work for both men and women
   6. Fair and Accurate Credit Transactions Act of 2003 (FACT)
      - Defines information that can be disclosed for credit history transactions (credit bureaus)
   7. Fair Credit Reporting Act of 1969
      - Discloses and makes understandable the workings of credit bureau processes
   8. Fair Labor Standards Act of 1938
      - Established minimum wages, overtime pay, recordkeeping, child labor laws, etc.
   9. Federal Insurance Contributions Act of 1935 (FICA) (Social Security)
      - Established the Social Security system
   10. Health Insurance Portability and Accountability Act (HIPAA) of 1996 (if company offers benefits)
       - Defines privacy in medical information and portability of plans
   11. Immigration Reform and Control Act of 1986
       - Made it illegal to knowingly hire illegal aliens
       - Employers must attest to immigration status
       - Gave immunity to illegal immigrants in the country before 1/1/1982
   12. National Labor Relations Act of 1947
       - Established right to form unions, strike, etc.
   13. Newborns' and Mothers' Health Protection Act of 1996
       - If plan offers maternity coverage, must pay minimum of 48 hours for childbirth (96 hours if C-section)
   14. Occupational Safety and Health Act (OSHA) of 1970
       - Defined work-related injury and safety regulations
   15. Sarbanes-Oxley Act of 2002

- Accountability of publicly held company boards, management, and public accounting firms (result of Enron-type issues)

16. Uniform Guidelines on Employee Selection Procedures of 1978
    - Defines legal tests and procedures for hiring
17. Uniformed Services Employment and Reemployment Rights Act of 1994
    - Establishes rights of military personnel to keep jobs while in service

B. For 11–14 employees, add

1. OSHA recordkeeping (maintain record of job-related injuries and illnesses)

C. For 15–19 employees, add

1. Title VII of the Civil Rights Act of 1964
    - See A.1 above
2. Americans with Disabilities Act of 1990
    - Prohibits discrimination based on disability

D. For 20–49 employees, add

1. Age Discrimination in Employment Act of 1967
    - Prohibits discrimination for hiring, promotion, etc., for those over age 40
2. Consolidated Omnibus Benefits Reconciliation Act (COBRA) of 1986
    - Allows for health benefits to be continued after leaving an employer

E. For 50–99 employees, add

1. Family and Medical Leave Act of 1993
    - Provides for time off in event of serious illness or birth of a child (both spouses)
2. EEO-1 Report (Equal Employment Opportunity) filed annually w/EEOC (Equal Employment Opportunity Commission) if organization is a federal contractor
    - Statically report on race/gender in company
3. Mental Health Parity Act of 1996 (for employers who offer mental health benefits)
    - Provides mental health benefits on parity with medical/surgical benefits

F. For 100 or more employees, add

1. Worker Adjustment and Retraining Notification Act of 1988
    - 60-day notice in the event of closing
2. EEO-1 Report filed annually w/EEOC if organization is not a federal contractor

G. Other items to be aware of

1. Employment law for managers
2. Harassment policies
3. Drug and alcohol issues
4. Worker's compensation
5. Unemployment insurance
6. Wage and hours laws

CHART 5.1 New employee orientation/annual competence checklist.

Employee Name: ____________________ **Signature:** ____________________
Reviewer Name: ____________________ **Signature:** ____________________
Date Reviewed: ____________________

	Competent	Reviewed by	Date
a. Answers phone promptly, appropriately; pleasant phone etiquette			
b. Patient scheduling performed appropriately/ accurately			
c. Knowledge of patient prep instructions/ documentation			
d. Competent at scheduling a CT exam—scheduler			
e. Competent at scheduling an XR exam—scheduler			
f. Competent at scheduling a MM exam—scheduler			
g. Competent at scheduling an US exam—scheduler			
h. Competent at scheduling an MR exam—scheduler			
i. Competent at scheduling an NM exam—scheduler			
j. Able to access and view the scheduling module			
k. Competent at checking out patient films to an outside facility—all			
I. Competent at checking in patient films to our facility—clerks			
m. Competent at preparing/processing overread exams to be read—all			
n. Competent at preparing/processing film comparison studies to be read—all			
o. Competent at reviewing patient profile and previous exams—all			
p. Obtains appropriate reports when necessary for a physician			
q. Makes sure all reports are in chronological order with most recent in front (MM)			
r. Knows where to get the scheduling office and the film library keys			
s. Knows what to do with the control (order sheet)			
t. Knows the different colors for OP/ER/Stats jackets			
u. Knows what to do with the call results—pink insert			
v. Knows where to put the signed consent forms to go to medical records			
w. Knows what to do with the outpatient's paperwork			
x. Knows where to find the outpatient's orders for patients			

(continued)

	Competent	Reviewed by	Date
Patients Coming to Imaging Services			
a. Greets all customers promptly and pleasantly upon arrival to department			
b. Attends to patient needs promptly and appropriately			
c. Obtains provider orders and checks immediately for accuracy			
d. Provides any consent/documentation for exam to be performed			
e. Confirms the patient has completed appropriate prep for exam—tech			
f. Knows how to order exams in HIS			
Film Library			
a. Obtains appropriate film jacket for comparison (MM, US, & MRI)			
b. Knows how to burn a CD from PACS			
c. Knows how to complete the film checkout—for films and CD			
Department Skills			
a. Proficient in the HIS systems			
b. Knows the PACS system			
c. Knowledge of digitizer for PACS			
d. Knowledgeable of server and desktop operating systems and databases			
e. Knowledgeable of interfaces used			
f. Facilitates the workflows and processes of the PACS including dailys			
g. Provide leadership and educate caregivers with the PACS system			
h. Serves as a resource for the institutional enterprise for physicians and caregivers			
i. Works with physicians and vendors			
j. Assists in ensuring HIPAA compliance			
k. Able to change patient status to "no show" in the HIS scheduling module			
Office Equipment			
a. Fax			
b. Copier			
c. Label printer			
d. Requisition printer			
e. Laser printers			
f. HIS monitors			
g. Department PC			

(continued)

	Competent	Reviewed by	Date
h. Teleradiology			
i. Takes items to be mailed to purchasing			
Knows Location of Manuals			
a. Housewide clinical policy and procedure manual			
b. MSDS manual			
c. Personnel manual			
d. Disaster plan			
e. Pharmacy formulary			
f. Exposure control/infection control manual			
g. Department manuals			
All			
a. Time sheets			
b. Bulletin boards/notices			
c. Parking			
d. Department organization charting and chain of command			
e. Hospital policies and procedures			
g. Employee policies and procedures			
h. Infection control policies and procedures			
i. Exposure control policies and procedures			
j. Material safety data sheets			
k. Disaster preparedness			
l. Fire plan—pull boxes and extinguisher locations			
m. Safety policies			
n. Guest relations			
o. Risk management/occurrence reporting			
p. Employee health/accident reporting			
q. Performance improvement			
r. Crash cart applications and protocol			
s. Pregnancy policy—patients			
t. Pregnancy policy—employee			
u. Informed consent—be able to print and fill out			
v. Nonionic contrast—be able to print and fill out			
w. Personnel dosimetry			
x. Cross-training			
y. Exam prioritization			
z. Other assigned responsibilities			
aa. Transportation policies and procedures			
bb. Protocols located for department you work in			
cc. Know how to access the intranet hospital policies			
dd. Know how to access the call schedule on the intranet			
ee. Spill kit—knows the location and has read the spill kit on educational site			

(continued)

	Competent	Reviewed by	Date
ff. Ticket to ride (patient transport handoff document)			
gg. Knows where the crash cart is located			
Orientation Checklist			
a. Call back and back up of personnel—where it is located and how to call tech in			
b. Holiday and shift coverage rotation			
c. Sick leave policy—has read the hospital intranet policy			
d. PTO requests—has read the hospital intranet policy			
e. Overtime policy and procedure—has read the hospital intranet policy			
f. Code/name tag—has read the hospital intranet policy			
g. Use of telephone and intercom system—has read the hospital intranet policy			
Customer Services			
a. Speaks courteously and respectfully to all customers and caregivers			
b. Consistently exhibits appropriate phone protocols			
c. Consistently displays cheerful and positive attitude			
d. Follows the chain of command in interdepartmental communication			
Patient Information Documentation			
a. Tech impression included in image set with history			
b. Communicates all appropriate information verbally and written to radiologist			
c. Obtains patient consent for all special procedures			
d. Able to put the comments for each patient in HIS			
e. Able to document in PACS for each patient in the internal notes section			
f. Enters patient into HIS system promptly and accurately when necessary			
g. Enters patient information into PACS for internal notes			
Patient Assessment			
a. Verification of procedure with physician order			
b. Checks for ID bracelet with request for proper identification			
c. Has patient or family member verify identity against the requisition			

(continued)

	Competent	Reviewed by	Date
d. Assesses physical condition of patient through observation			
e. Verifies preparation instructions were followed by patient before the procedure			
f. Checks exam request for mode of transport and additional needs			
g. Assesses physical condition of patient prior to transporting			
h. Consults with patient/nurse/radiologist when appropriate regarding exam			
i. Patient's safety and comfort monitored and acted upon throughout exam			
Professional Ethics and Attitude			
a. Transports patient appropriately			
b. Shows respect for patient modesty			
c. Applies patient comfort procedures			
d. Accepts constructive criticism			
e. Shows ability to adapt to new situations			
f. Instills confidence in the patient			
g. Explains the exam to the patient before and during procedure			
h. Exhibits appropriate patient communication			
i. Exhibits the self-confidence to perform the procedure			
j. Uses proper infection control precautions			
k. Respects patient rights to confidentiality			
l. Communicates post procedure instructions to patient			

Employee Comments:

Employee Action/Self-Development Plan:

Note:

6 Evaluation, Appraisal, Retention, and Dismissal

EVALUATION AND APPRAISAL

Formal evaluation and performance appraisal should be performed at minimum on an annual basis. Confidentiality must be ensured. Expectations should be known and agreed to by both employee and management. The appraisal should be no surprise to either.

Evaluation forms should be used to document the process. The frequency of evaluation should be set, as stated, at least annually. Some institutions use a midyear coaching tool to ensure an employee's progress. Personnel files should be kept on all employees. In legal situations (claims against the employer, etc.), this is the most pivotal piece of evidence. It also should be used to document accomplishments.

Having documented ongoing performance helps to avoid the *halo effect*, where most recent behaviors (good or bad) influence the appraisal process.

Input should be sought from others regarding performance. These can be peers, physicians, and others working in the department. Toward the end of the process, mutually agreeable goals should be set for the coming period, utilizing the employee's input. Extra reward should be established for "stretch" goals—those that excel.

Career development plans should be a factor when appropriate. Recognition for accomplishments should be also documented

Documents should be signed by management and staff. An employee signs to *acknowledge receiving* the document, not necessarily for the purpose of *agreeing with* the appraisal (Table 6.1).

RETENTION

Large amounts of resources are expended in the interview, hiring, and orientation process. It is therefore wise to have a plan to retain as many good caregivers as possible.

Eventually, the competition for human resources will increase in the medical imaging field. This will be due to a variety of factors including the aging baby boomers, increasing regulatory requirements requiring more time and human resources to comply, and a host of other reasons.

Because retention is the final goal of the whole process, an effective screening process during the interview and hiring phase is necessary.

TABLE 6.1
Sample Evaluation Form

DATE:

CAREGIVER SIGNATURE:

EVAL TYPE: ☐ Annual ☐ 3 month ☐ Other

EVALUATION SCORING SYSTEM

5	*Exceptional*	*90%–100%*
4	*Frequently Exceeds Standard*	*80%–89%*
3	*Competent, meets standard*	*60%–79%*
2	*Needs Improvement*	*40%–59%*
1	*Unacceptable Performance*	*1%–39%*

QUALITY: Applies the standard of practice/performance in full work setting to achieve positive outcomes.

Check all that apply to the scope of patient care services

Infant	0–1 year
Pediatric	13 months–12 years
Adolescent	13 years–17 years
Adult	18 years–64 years
Older Adult	65 years +

RATING SUPERVISOR	DATE
DEPARTMENT HEAD	DATE
ADMINISTRATION	DATE
HUMAN RESOURCES	DATE

MISSION:

VISION:

Caregiver Name ______________________ Job Title ______________________

All caregivers are expected to consistently exhibit organizational core values. Core values serve to define and support the determination of a numerical rating based on percentage of time a caregiver exhibits the behavior.

Criteria Specific to Organizational Values

(* column is for director rating, as needed)

Integrity: Upholding a high level of ethics, morals and values	**EX**	**FE**	**C**	**NI**	**U**	*
As evidenced by, for example:	**5**	**4**	**3**	**2**	**1**	
* Adheres to dress code; appearance is neat and clean; wears identification badge while on duty						
* Responsible and accountable for own individual behavior						
* Protects confidential information at all times						
* Upholds the standards of individual ethical and legal business practices						
Compassion: Recognizing and addressing customer concerns	**EX**	**FE**	**C**	**NI**	**U**	*
As evidenced by, for example:	**5**	**4**	**3**	**2**	**1**	
* Creates a caring and comfortable environment for patients, families, friends, physicians, and staff						
* Is present body, mind, and spirit for anyone in need						
* Is aware of customers' concerns and goes out of his or her way to assist						
Accountability: Holding self accountable to the quality of his/her work	**EX**	**FE**	**C**	**NI**	**U**	*
As evidenced by, for example:	**5**	**4**	**3**	**2**	**1**	
*Taking an obligation or willingness to accept responsibility and/or ownership of one's actions or nonactions						
*Following through with established goals						
*Communicates work plan status and seeks clarification of goals/methods as necessary						
Respect: Appreciating customer needs and responding to them	**EX**	**FE**	**C**	**NI**	**U**	*
As evidenced by, for example:	**5**	**4**	**3**	**2**	**1**	
* Recognizes and communicates the worth and importance of each person with whom he or she interacts						
* Promotes and demonstrates respect, honesty, and straightforwardness in daily work activities						
* Relates to all customers with a friendly, caring, and helpful attitude						
* Treats others as we would want ourselves or our loved ones to be treated (i.e., with courtesy, compassion, respect)						

(continued)

TABLE 6.1 (CONTINUED)
Sample Evaluation Form

		EX	FE	C	NI	U	*
Excellence: Striving to be the best		**EX**	**FE**	**C**	**NI**	**U**	*
	As evidenced by, for example:	**5**	**4**	**3**	**2**	**1**	
	* Acknowledges and accepts change based on mission, vision, and values of the organization						
	* Pursues personal improvement in ways that enhance quality of job performance and service to customers						
	* Maintains a willingness to work as part of a team, promotes positive relationships within and between departments, takes an active role in the improvement process						
Behavioral Standards		**EX**	**FE**	**C**	**NI**	**U**	*
1	*Courtesy: treats the people we serve as guests	5	4	3	2	1	
2	*Professional Image: presents self with a professional image	5	4	3	2	1	
3	*Telephone: answers the phone with a smile	5	4	3	2	1	
4	*Listen and Clarify: listens to requests and responds appropriately	5	4	3	2	1	
5	*How Can I Help? anticipates the wants and needs of those we serve	5	4	3	2	1	
6	*Communication: communicates with patient's families and co-workers effectively	5	4	3	2	1	
7	*Keep Them Informed: keeps those we serve informed about their care and treatment	5	4	3	2	1	
8	*Safety and Cleanliness: maintains a safe and clean environment	5	4	3	2	1	
9	*4-A Process: anticipates, acknowledges, apologizes, and amends negative service situations	5	4	3	2	1	
10	*Master the Skills: strives to master the skills needed to do your best for the people we serve	5	4	3	2	1	
11	*Positive Representation: positively represents hospital in the workplace and the community	5	4	3	2	1	
12	*Teamwork: strives to be a team player departmentally and organizationally	5	4	3	2	1	
13	*Attitude: presents self with a positive, compassionate, and caring attitude	5	4	3	2	1	
14	*Commitment to Co-workers: shows workforce commitment to co-workers	5	4	3	2	1	
15	*Accountability: holds self accountable to the quality of his/her work	5	4	3	2	1	

SUMMARY

1. What accomplishments have you achieved this year?
2. What are your work strengths?
3. What are your opportunities for improvement?
4. What would you like to accomplish during the next evaluation period?
5. How will these accomplishments support the mission and values of the regional medical center?

Supervisor Comments:

Caregiver's Comments:

Total Points ______ divided by total points possible ______ = ______ × 100 = ______ Overall Rating: ______

If caregiver's overall score is *Needs Improvement* or *Unacceptable Performance* an employee improvement action plan must be attached.

Note: Scoring system; EX: Exceptional; FE: Frequently exceeds standards; C: Competent, meets standards; NI: Needs improvement; U: Unacceptable performance.

What is most important to employees is *not* salary or benefits—it is *personal worth, achievement, and appreciation.* Employees typically leave a position because of issues with their direct supervisor. To keep this from occurring, the following should be set forth:

- Make expectations clear.
- Provide regular feedback.
- Keep employees in the loop where appropriate.
- Obtain employee input.

Motivation, salary, and benefits can help to retain employees. Make sure to work with the human resources department to ensure the institution is competitive.

Minimizing stress on the job can help to keep good caregivers.

When possible the institution should establish career ladders that will give employees a chance for advancement.

DISMISSAL

Having to dismiss a caregiver is one of the most uncomfortable tasks a manager will have to perform. Typically, the orientation period is used to assess competency. If possible, consider suspension before dismissal.

If termination is necessary, terminate a caregiver before too much damage occurs (influencing other employees negatively, etc.).

A *progressive disciplinary* procedure must have occurred. This usually consists of a verbal warning, written warning, and then termination. The time frame for these steps varies by institution.

Issues must be documented and discussed with the caregiver. Consider using a *termination checklist* so nothing is missed. The caregiver must be given a chance to improve. It can be helpful to construct an improvement plan with parameters and timelines with the caregiver.

Many institutions will conduct an exit interview. It is vital that more than one company person be present during this procedure.

There are many legal ramifications involved in dismissal, so make sure a human resources expert is consulted during the termination process.

It must be emphasized to the caregiver that work behavior is the issue, *not* the person.

After terminating an employee, future reference requests for the former employee should state only the position and dates of employment.

Section III

Operations Management

7 Department Planning
Layout and Design

Department design and layout can be put into two categories: new areas and redesign. The best way to structure this process is to use project management.

The first part of project management is to choose who will be on the team. Depending on the scope of the project, you will want to include the planners—architects, radiologists, administrators, staff, and clerical staff. Many architectural firms specialize in the planning of imaging departments.

After you have determined who will be on the team, you will want to designate a point person who will facilitate communications between the department and architects, hospital planners, contractors, and so forth.

All members of the team should participate in the establishment of timelines for planning, construction, and opening.

The next important step is to develop a communication plan for your department and all other departments and users that may or will be impacted by some phase of your construction or renovation.

Workflow must be optimized, for both radiologists and staff. In addition, patient flow and waiting areas must be taken into consideration.

Will there be new technology that will impact space or workflow? This will make it important to put space aside for expansion (or contraction, in the case of diminishing darkrooms).

A typical imaging department consists of the following components:

- Inner/outer corridors—outer corridors are typically public/patient areas, whereas inner corridors are for staff
- Inpatient/outpatient areas should be separate, and separate waiting/changing areas when possible
  - Separate male/female waiting/changing areas
- Patient holding areas
- Women's specialty studies
  - Ultrasound, breast procedures
- Patient interview areas
  - Confidentiality important
- Financial counseling in department if possible

INFRASTRUCTURE

Infrastructure areas are all of those that need to be considered in department layout. Standard square footage and locations can be determined by an architect. These include but are not limited to the following:

- Information technology
- Picture archiving and communication system (PACS)
- Radiology information system (RIS)
- CR (computed radiography) DR (direct radiography)
- All specialty areas:
  - MRI
  - CT
  - PET
  - Nuclear medicine
    - Hot lab requirements, ventilation, etc.
- Ultrasound
- Teleradiology consulting area
- Electrical needs
- Lighting
- Communications—overhead, etc.
- Plumbing—darkroom (if needed)
- QC (quality control) areas—location of PACS monitors, RIS components
- Reading areas
- Scheduling/reception
- Consulting areas (physician)
- Reference library
- File room (plus archival studies)
- Transcription
- Storage
- Administration
- Break area
- Staff rooms
- ADA (Americans with Disabilities Act) restrooms
- Janitor closets

HIPAA COMPLIANCE

An important consideration in planning is compliance with the Health Insurance Portability and Accountability Act (HIPAA). HIPAA regulations include considerations for patient privacy:

- Visual—can patients see computer screens or scheduling boards?
- Audible—can patients overhear other patients who are being asked to provide information? This often occurs in combined reception and waiting areas.

SUPPLIES

Supply acquisition and storage is another space-planning consideration.

- Where will supply deliveries come in?
- Where will supplies and linens be stored until they can be put away?
- Is there adequate supply storage?
- Is storage conveniently close so that staff do not have to travel long distances for often-used items?

OTHER ARCHITECTURAL CONSIDERATIONS

- Ceiling mounted tubes—can ceiling support the weight?
- Floor load—especially CT and MR
- Hookups for gases and suction
- Cable needs—CR, DR, PACS, computers, printers
- Adjacent space for future growth
- What is above and below the exam room?
- What is the acuity of patients you will serve?
    - ICU patients in beds require more space than outpatients.
- Will you need pre- or post-procedure areas?
- What is the maximum number of staff you could expect to be in a room at one time?

These are all considerations as room space is determined.

EXAM ROOM DETERMINATION

There are various methods to determine the number of needed radiographic rooms. One is as follows:

1. Multiply annual procedure volume by the average procedure time in minutes.
2. Subtract the procedure minutes from the total available minutes.
3. Utilization of 80% would suggest the need for an additional room.

EXAM ROOM UTILIZATION EXAMPLE

- 5,000 procedures × average procedure time of 15 min = 75,000 min
- 8 hours × 60 min × 5 days × 50 weeks = 120,000
- 120,000 min – 75,000 min = 45,000 min
- 45,000/120,000 = 37.5%
- Room utilization = 62.5%

Room/Equipment Capacity and Type

Items to consider when calculating rooms and capacity.

- Vendors have typical capacities by modality
- Space calculations
- Square foot determinations decided by common formulas that architects utilize
- Hallway/door widths
- Lead lining/magnetic shielding (up to 8 feet high)
    - Determined by modality
    - Lead lining possibly needed (low dosage)—depends on composition of wall material and areas surrounding room
- Radiographic/interventional/CT/dedicated chest
- Mammographic
- Stereotactic breast biopsy rooms
- Bone densitometry
- Nuclear medicine
- Magnetic shielding
- MRI

WORKFLOW

Workflow in the medical imaging department has changed dramatically with the advent of computers and digital imaging. Changes with the advent of RIS/PACS/CR/DR have changed equipment and workflow.

With this in mind, planning should consider workstation locations and numbers. Radiologists will need to have areas that are quiet and dark just as when reading standard films. In addition, there has to be easy access and room for consulting with referring physicians.

Traffic flow should be traced from several perspectives:

- Inpatient flow
- Outpatient flow
- Technologist flow
- Radiologist flow
- Clerical flow
- Reception flow

When possible, strategically locate patient routes to and from exam areas.

Also to be considered are specific specialty areas, such as women's imaging.

It is important to plan so that patients are in sight at all times by a staff member.

Plan patient tracking points if a patient tracking function on the department computer system will be utilized (RIS function).

8 Staffing

Staffing is probably one of the most difficult tasks a new manager can tackle. Covering different modalities, different shifts, call, and so forth can be daunting. Associated personnel issues also come into play—sick call-in, vacation, medical leave, and others.

The first step is to determine the amount of staffing needed and the times or shifts that need to be covered.

Staffing ratios have been collected, but no optimal ratio can be projected. Accrediting agencies and payer entities also indirectly affect staffing through phrases like *optimal patient care*. Staffing is also one of the most expensive areas in an imaging department. Effects like *burnout* also have to be monitored. Historically there has been a cyclical nature of technologist shortages. This has varied by modality. Imaging technologist schools will turn out graduates no matter what the job market is, because they realize a profit from having students. Recent economic conditions have compelled many people to return to school for a different career. This has attracted many new students. Technology reduces the necessity of caregivers in some areas (clerical, film room) and increases the need in others (computer-driven areas like information technology, picture archiving and communication system [PACS], radiology information system [RIS], etc.). Relatively new modalities such as bone densitometry, positron emission tomography (PET), PET/computed tomography (CT), molecular imaging, and others require new caregiver training.

Regulations that limit the types of personnel necessary to perform exams can change demand. Many states do not require an x-ray technologist to be registered.

Specialty accreditations such as magnetic resonance imaging (MRI) and CT require that technologists in those areas be registered or certified. This requires extra training. Accreditation requires a minimal number of exams to be done before the candidate can sit for the specialty exam. Many times this will require double coverage in a modality while training occurs.

Some payers (particularly Medicare, which now accounts for a minimum of about 50% of revenue in most institutions) require that technologists performing the exams be registered/certified in order for the institution to be paid for performing those exams.

AMERICAN REGISTRY OF RADIOLOGIC TECHNOLOGISTS' 12 POST-PRIMARY QUALIFICATIONS

- Bone Densitometry (BD)
- Breast Sonography (BS)
- Cardiovascular Interventional Radiography (Note: No longer available for new candidates)

- Cardiac Interventional Radiography (CI)
- Computed Tomography (CT)
- Magnetic Resonance Imaging (MRI) (Primary and Post-Primary Tracks)
- Mammography (M)
- Quality Management (QM)
- Sonography (S) (Primary and Post-Primary Tracks)
- Vascular Sonography (VS)
- Vascular Interventional Technology (VI)
- Registered Radiologist Assistant (RRA, new in September 2005)

WHAT CAN IMPACT STAFFING

Besides normal shift staffing, a variety of factors can also have an impact such as the following:

- New services
- New service lines
- New technology—PACS, RIS
- New programs startups
- New procedures
- New physicians
- Expansion of services in the operating room or emergency department
- Change in procedure volumes
- Modality migration
- Elimination of service or service lines
- Student programs
- Reduction in workforce

Cross-Training

One of the solutions to staffing issues can be cross-training.

- Advantages:
  - Staff able to work in more than one modality or specialty area
  - Opportunity for career growth
  - Can reduce the number of staff needed
  - Works best in small or low-volume departments
- Disadvantages:
  - Staff often want to only work in the specialty area
  - Difficult to keep staff skills at the needed level if there is not a regular rotation in all areas
- Busy and/or high-volume departments need the cross-trained staff at the same times

On Demand

In many ways, staffing in medical imaging is unlike any other business, including staffing in other areas of a healthcare institution. Imaging is partially an *on-demand* department, which means that in addition to the scheduled exams, there are walk-in patients and emergency patients. Also, imaging is a 24/7 department. This makes staffing a very complex process, which requires integrating a variety of factors.

Most of the heavy workload is during the day, when both inpatient and outpatient care is provided. In an outpatient (nonhospital) setting, most referrals come during the normal working day. However, recently many outpatient entities have begun offering extended hours for patients that need to have studies done after work.

The number of staff depends on typical demand. Various other departments will feed patients into imaging. One of the first steps to be taken is to analyze the data that represents exam volume by hour and type. This data can usually be extracted from the information system being utilized.

Chart 8.1 demonstrates total volume by hour. Several points are of interest:

- Volumes gradually increase as the morning progresses.
- Volumes peak during the noon hour.
- Volume decline slightly, and then go up at the end of the day.
- After 5 p.m., volumes decline as expected. Studies done in the late evening and very early morning are probably portables from the ICU or emergency room studies.

Looking at the data, the manager should try to figure out why volumes peak at certain times to appropriate staff. What was discovered in this situation is that the midmorning peak is normal and expected. This is when most contrast studies are done because patients are fasting the night before. However, what the manager also

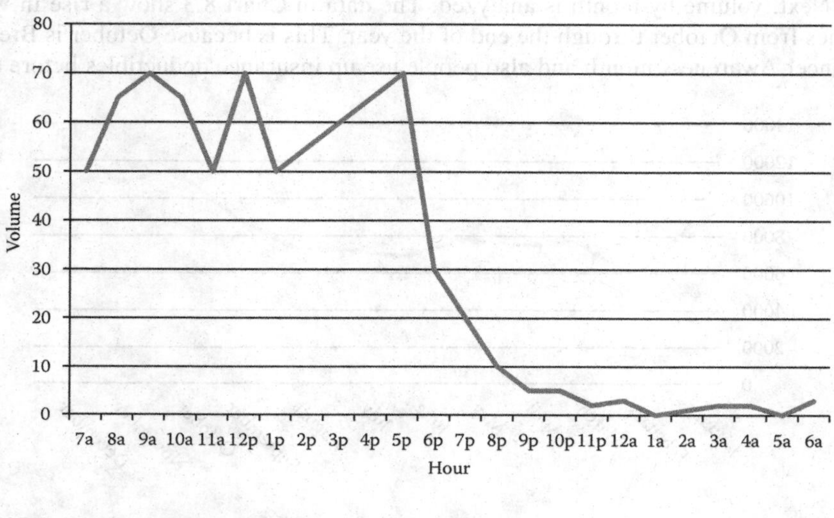

CHART 8.1 Exam volume by hour of the day.

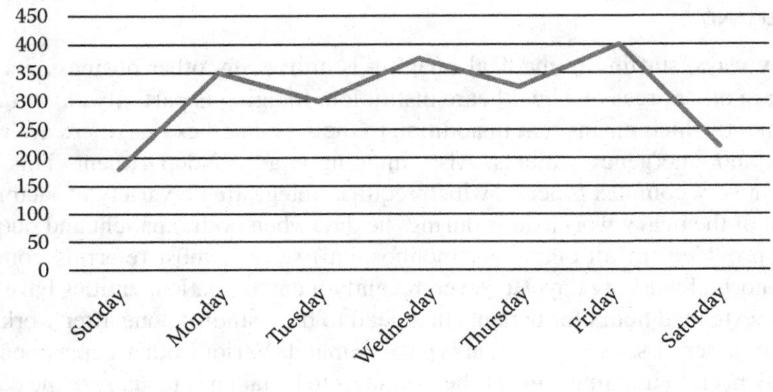

CHART 8.2 Exam volume by day of the week.

discovered is that the orthopedic clinic sees patients all morning, orders x-ray studies, and then breaks for lunch. The orthopedic department assumes that these studies can all be completed and results will be ready when the orthopedic doctors get back from lunch. The challenge the manager has now is to get the studies completed in a timely manner while allowing his or her own staff lunch time.

The next set of data to be reviewed is volume demand by days of the week. Chart 8.2 demonstrates this. Several points are of interest:

- Volumes are relatively steady Monday through Thursday.
- Volumes peak on Fridays.

What is discovered here is that the emergency room sends most of the patients in the evening on Friday.

Next, volume by month is analyzed. The data in Chart 8.3 show a rise in volumes from October through the end of the year. This is because October is Breast Cancer Awareness month and also people use up insurance deductibles before the

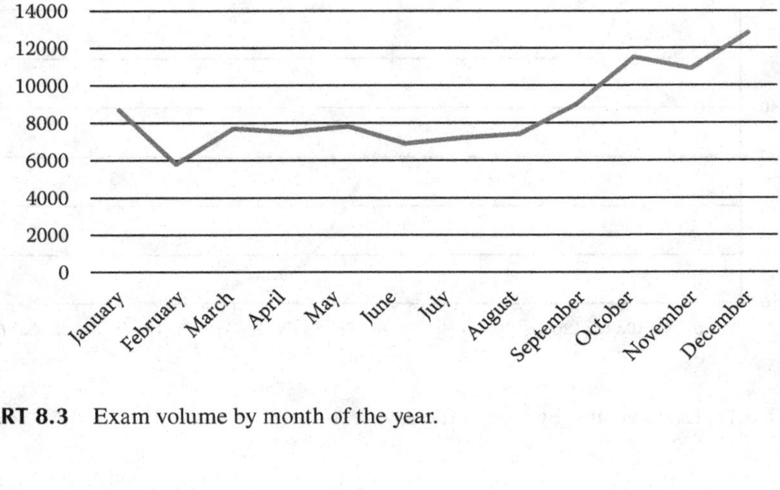

CHART 8.3 Exam volume by month of the year.

end of the year. Women typically try to book mammograms during October, but many cannot get appointments, so these volumes spill over into November and December.

Modality

The above analysis demonstrates a sample of how data should be utilized to predict staffing. The same type of analysis should be done by individual *modality*. A modality in medical imaging is an individual area such as CT, MRI, nuclear medicine, ultrasound, and so forth.

Emergency room referrals should be tracked by volume, modality, and hour. Referrals from high utilizers, such as orthopedics, should also be considered. Orthopedic studies are typically manpower intensive, as they can sometimes involve exotic views and patient conditions.

Outpatient clinic volumes sent to imaging have defined hours and can be more easily projected.

One often-overlooked parameter involved in staffing considerations is the availability and number of radiologists, radiology residents (if the facility has a residency program), and radiology PAs (physician assistants) on staff. If there is a high workload of exams involving them but few radiologists to cover them, numbers of technologists and technologist extenders can be reduced. Radiology residents can perform a high volume of exams. Conversely, teaching residents also reduces the radiologist's productivity.

Lunch and break coverage and sick and vacation coverage must also be considered. Approving vacation requests should factor in the time of year. The best scenario is to allow vacations during the slowest months of the year. Sick time is harder to predict. However, historical data can help. Sick days usually peak during flu season, as one would expect.

Family Medical Leave Act

The Family Medical Leave Act mandates up to six weeks off for certain situations, such as the birth of a child. Employees utilizing this time off can adversely affect staffing in the short and long run. Their position must be the same level and number of hours when they return from leave.

ENSURING ADEQUATE STAFF COVERAGE

After volume demands are determined, several different methods can be effective to ensure proper coverage. One such method is *staggered scheduling*, where shift start and end times are staggered. This ensures coverage during the most heavy workload periods and smooth crossover during shift changes.

The next consideration is *staffing levels by modality*. Typically, these modalities are the following:

- Mammography
- CT
- Ultrasound
- MRI
- PET
- Nuclear Medicine
- Bone Densitometry
- Angiography/Special Procedures

Some institutions have technologist training programs, and the student help needs to be considered. First-year students can do some procedures by the end of the first year, but they typically reduce productivity for the technologist doing the training because of the inherent teaching element.

The next element to be considered is *support staff*, which usually includes the following:

- Registration
- Scheduling
- Transport aides
- PACS/RIS support personnel
- File room
- Clerical
- Radiology aides
- Administration

In addition, if the facility decides to add new services or service lines, such as women's services (mammography, stereotactic breast biopsy, breast ultrasound, etc.), the staffing implications must be considered.

The addition of new technology will also impact staffing. The addition of PACS, for instance, can increase or decrease staffing depending on how it is utilized. Another example would be if the radiologists decided to start their own nighthawk or dayhawk service. There are associated exams and documents that add to the department's workload.

In summation, the major considerations for determining staffing levels consist of

- Types of exams performed (modalities)
- Number of technologists/aides necessary by modality
- Hours of day exams offered
- Wait time necessary for exams requiring a radiologist
- New service lines
- New technology

To illustrate various scenarios, an example will be considered. See box below.

Another solution is to have the technologists *cross-trained* so that they are capable of performing exams in more than one modality. As an example, a second-shift technologist may be trained in x-ray and crossed-trained in CT. Care must be taken

EXAMPLE

CT SCANNING

- Typical eight-hour day: one exam = 45 minutes
- Allow time for processing, radiologist review, patient/room preparation
- Keep flexible for add-ons: ER, others
- Determine time needed for different exam types
- Allow time for retakes, additional views requested by radiologist, special considerations (isolation, MRSA, AIDS patients, etc.), post-processing, and other situations

STAFFING SCENARIO A

- 1 CT tech = 1 exam/hour
- 45-minute exam time, 15-minute prep + room clean time between patients
- Results in 8 exams/day

RADIOLOGY EXTENDERS

Staffing can be significantly improved using *radiology extenders*. These people are compensated at a lower level than technologists, and they do not perform the exam. They assist with the duties that need to be done but not necessarily by technologists. They reduce tech time for nonessential duties such as patient interview, patient prep and transport, contrast prep, cleanup, study/jacket retrieval, and others.

STAFFING SCENARIO B

- 1 CT tech, 1 aide
- 45-minute exam time, back to back
- 45-minute exams × 8 hours = 10.6 exams/day

Some facilities use 2 CT techs per room. This has shown to increase the number of exams per day.

to consider what happens when the emergency room sends more than one patient to imaging at about the same time that requires different modality exams.

A cross-trained individual is usually compensated at a higher level than a single-modality-trained technologist. These individuals are highly valuable when there is a shortage of qualified individuals in the market.

Flexible staffing can be employed. This allows a staff person to leave if volumes for the day are down and the department is slow.

Staffing Ratios and Full-Time Equivalents

The manager could use historical *staffing ratios*, such as examinations per full-time equivalent (FTE) technologist, equal to 52 weeks times 40 hours per week, or 2,080 hours. Further numerical determination of FTEs will be covered in Chapter 14. Historical ratios should always be used in conjunction with actual present and predicted needs. The staffing budget will help determine projected number and types of exams, which in turn will drive staffing needs.

It is important to remember there is a baseline staff that will be present regardless of the projected workload.

EXTERNAL FACTORS AFFECTING STAFFING

Aging of the Baby Boomers

The baby boomers are gradually aging and will require a large increase in healthcare, which includes imaging studies.

By the year 2030—

- The over-65 population will nearly double.
- More than 6 of every 10 boomers will be managing more than one chronic condition.
- More than 1 out of every 3 boomers—over 10 million—will be considered obese.
- One out of every 4 boomers—over 14 million—will be living with diabetes.
- Nearly 1 out of every 2 boomers—more than 26 million—will be living with arthritis.
- Eight times more knee replacements will be performed than are performed today.

The impact on the healthcare system is obvious.

Public Awareness

For several years there has been an increasing awareness of healthcare issues by the general public. Technologists have historically had to answer questions about radiation doses and safety. With the increases in public awareness, it is more important than ever that staff are certified in their specialty.

Specialty Certifications

At present, there are 5 primary certifications and 11 subspecialty certifications:

- *Primary*—Radiography (R), Nuclear Medicine (N), Radiation Therapy (T), Sonography (S), and Magnetic Resonance Imaging (MRI)

- *Subspecialty*—Quality Management (QM), Vascular Sonography (VS), Cardiac Interventional Radiography (CI), Bone Densitometry (BD), Breast Sonography (BS), Computed Tomography (CT), Sonography (S), Magnetic Resonance Imaging (MRI), Registered Radiology Assistant (RRA), Mammography (M), and Vascular Interventional Technologist (VI)

Staffing shortages typically occur in cycles. For a few years, there was a shortage of sonographers and an oversupply of nuclear medicine technologists. Partially because of the advent of PET/CT, nuclear medicine has enjoyed a recent resurgence. It is wise to read publications in the industry to ascertain coming shortages, when they are possible to predict.

Accreditations

Medicare has recently mandated *accreditation* for imaging. What this means is that an imaging department must go through a rigorous process for equipment and staff to receive approval. There are several accrediting agencies. The most prominent are the ACR (American College of Radiology) and the IAC (Intersocietal Accreditation Commission). Other large healthcare payers are following suit and also mandating accreditations.

Limited Licensure

State laws vary requiring accreditation (see Table 8.1). Some states allow *limited licensure*, while others do not. Limited licensure allows technologists trained in only certain areas to only do exams in those areas.

Some states have no certification requirements at all. In these states, many small offices employ clerical personnel to do imaging studies. Mandatory accreditation will reduce the number of offices employing these practices.

As part of the accreditation process, the accrediting agencies require technologists to hold certification. In addition, certification has continuing education requirements after the certification has been achieved.

CARE Act

The CARE Act (Consistency, Accuracy, Responsibility, and Excellence in Medical Imaging and Radiation Therapy Act of 2007) intends to make imaging studies safer, less costly, and more accurate. This act impacts staffing ratios in a variety of ways. Making imaging studies less costly implies fewer staff per exam. Accuracy implies better studies the first time around, which implies better-trained, more-efficient personnel.

There are professional organizations that collect current staffing ratio data. The data are compared in a variety of ways. It is important to use this data as a guideline only, as most situations are unique (see Table 8.2).

Some staffing ratio information can be obtained from the following organizations:

- The American Healthcare Radiology Administrators, www.ahraonline.org
- The American College of Radiology, www.acr.org
- Aunt Minnie website, www.auntminnie.com

TABLE 8.1
Limited Licensure by State

State	No Requirement	Accept Ltd. License	ARRT Ltd. License	Ltd. Licensure Requirement
Arizona		Y		Limited licensure is granted by the board for state practical technologists who have completed a state-approved course that provides 210 hours of academic curriculum and 480 hours of clinical training. Students must participate in a limited license program in Arizona (no home-study or online courses) in order to obtain a limited license in x-ray.
Arkansas		Y	Y	The state also issues limited scope certification to those who successfully pass the ARRT limited scope examination. Students interested in obtaining Limited Scope Certification are not required to attend a formal school before taking the ARRT examination. However, the state board encourages students to take a course to prepare for the ARRT examination and recommends *Radiography Essentials for Limited Practice*, 2nd edition, available through the Radiation Board office.
Alabama	Y			
California		Y		The state also issues limited permits in x-ray. Limited permit applicants must have completed a course of study through an approved school in the state of California, as well as completion of a specific prescribed number of clinical exams (logs) at an approved clinical education site before they are eligible to take the state-administered limited license exam.

(continued)

TABLE 8.1 (CONTINUED)
Limited Licensure by State

State	No Requirement	Accept Ltd. License	ARRT Ltd. License	Ltd. Licensure Requirement
Colorado		Y	Y	Limited licensure is also permitted, and those individuals must demonstrate competency via satisfactory passage of a limited scope examination (75% or higher) administered by the American Registry of Radiologic Technologists (ARRT). Those wishing to obtain a limited scope license might consider preparing for the exam using the Glacier Valley Medical Education courses.
Connecticut		N		
Delaware		Y	Y	The state also issues limited scope certification to those who successfully pass the ARRT limited scope examination.
DC	Y			
Florida		Y		The Florida Office of Radiation Control issues licensure in Basic x-ray machine operator (BMO). At present, there is no minimum educational requirement to take the BMO certification examination. The Department of Health and Rehabilitative Services provides some study material upon initial application for the BMO certification examination.
Georgia	Y			
Hawaii		N		
Idaho	Y			
Illinois		Y	Y	The state also grants limited radiography licensure to those who prepare for and pass the ARRT limited scope examination.
Indiana		Y	Y	The state also grants limited certification to those who prepare for and pass the ARRT limited scope examination.

(continued)

TABLE 8.1 (CONTINUED)
Limited Licensure by State

State	No Requirement	Accept Ltd. License	ARRT Ltd. License	Ltd. Licensure Requirement
Iowa		Y	Y	The state also issues licensure to limited radiographers who complete a state-approved 100-hour training course and pass the ARRT limited radiography examination.
Kansas		Y		The state also issues licensure to radiographers who complete a state-approved limited license training course.
Kentucky		Y		Those individuals holding limited certification cannot be employed in a facility that utilizes contrast media. Students interested in obtaining limited certification must complete a limited radiography program that is approved by the state or an independent study course available from the Radiation Control Branch.
Louisiana		Y		You may meet the qualifications for certification as a private radiologic technologist as issued by the Louisiana Board of Medical Examiners (BME). The BME only has jurisdiction over persons employed by licensed physicians in that physician's own private offices.
Maine		Y		A limited radiographer is a person other than a licensed practitioner who applies x-radiation to specific parts of the human body for diagnostic purposes while under the supervision of a licensed practitioner. The categories of limited radiography are skull, spine, chest, extremities, and podiatry. No more than two categories shall be held by any limited license holder. Fluoroscopy is not permitted for limited permit holders. The individual must complete a state approved course prior to taking the state examination.
Maryland		N		

(continued)

TABLE 8.1 (CONTINUED)
Limited Licensure by State

State	No Requirement	Accept Ltd. License	ARRT Ltd. License	Ltd. Licensure Requirement
Massachusetts		Y		Noncertified radiologic technologists as defined in "Regulations Governing the Licensing of Radiologic Technologists for Massachusetts." An individual who is not certified as a radiologic technologist (ARRT) must complete a state-accredited program prior to taking the state limited scope exam.
Michigan	Y			
Minnesota		Y		X-ray operators (anyone who is not a radiologic technologist registered by the ARRT) are required to pass the state x-ray operators exam. There are currently three state-approved testing centers. Those who pass the x-ray operator examination are allowed to perform any x-ray examination that the facility where they are employed wishes them to do.
Mississippi		N		
Missouri		N		
Montana		Y		For radiologic technologist limited licensure, individuals must complete a state-approved 40-hour program. No prior experience is required. Currently, District 6 Health Care Learning Center in Billings offers the only state-approved limited licensure program, entitled Basic X-ray Techniques.
Nebraska		Y	Y	Individuals must pass the ARRT limited scope examination with a score of 75% or higher. The State Radiology Board of Nebraska encourages students to take a course to prepare for the examination.
Nevada	No except mammo			
New Hampshire	Y			

(continued)

TABLE 8.1 (CONTINUED)
Limited Licensure by State

State	No Requirement	Accept Ltd. License	ARRT Ltd. License	Ltd. Licensure Requirement
New Jersey		Y		Issues limited permits in radiography. Limited permit aspirants are required to submit a course completion certificate from a state-approved school before they can take the state licensure examination.
New Mexico		Y		Grants a certificate of limited practice to limited radiologic practitioners. To obtain a certificate, the student must attend a state-approved course.
New York		N		
North Carolina	Y			
North Dakota	Y			
Ohio		Y		The minimum requirement for any individual performing x-ray procedures in the state of Ohio is that the individual be licensed as a general x-ray machine operator. In order to obtain a license as a general x-ray machine operator, the applicant must attend an educational program accredited by the Ohio Department of Health. After completion of the approved program, the applicant must pass the state license examination.
Oklahoma	Y			
Oregon		Y		The state also issues limited permits in radiography. Limited permit aspirants are required to submit a course completion certificate from a state-approved school before they can take the Oregon state examination.
Pennsylvania		N		
Rhode Island		N		

(continued)

TABLE 8.1 (CONTINUED)
Limited Licensure by State

State	No Requirement	Accept Ltd. License	ARRT Ltd. License	Ltd. Licensure Requirement
South Carolina		Y		The state also issues certification for limited practice radiographers. Limited certification aspirants are required to submit a course completion certificate from a state-approved school before they can take the licensure examination.
South Dakota		Y		Any person who has 24 hours of orientation and training in the operation of radiation producing equipment by a qualified instructor may operate any radiation producing device.
Tennessee		Y		The state also issues limited certification in x-ray. The holder of a limited permit is enabled to perform only those radiological procedures or functions intended for the body areas indicated on the issued certification, other than those procedures involving the administration of contrast media. Limited certification is available in the following areas: chest, extremities, skull (AP and lateral only), sinuses, and lumbar spine (AP and lateral only). The individual must submit verification of attendance and successful completion of a state board–approved radiological certification training course for the type of certification sought pursuant to Rule 0880-50.05(2) and successfully complete the board-approved examination.
Texas		Y		The state also grants limited x-ray licensure to students who have completed a state-approved 8-month course.

(continued)

TABLE 8.1 (CONTINUED)
Limited Licensure by State

State	No Requirement	Accept Ltd. License	ARRT Ltd. License	Ltd. Licensure Requirement
Utah		Y		The state also grants licensure to radiology practical technicians in accordance with subsection 58-54-5(3). A practical technician must pass the Utah Limited Scope of Practice in Radiography Examination, administered by the professional licensing board.
Virginia		Y		The state also grants radiologic technologist limited licensure. Those individuals must complete a state-approved program as described in regulations 18 VAC 85-101-70.
Vermont		Y		The state also issues limited radiography licensure, with an endorsement for chest radiography, extremities radiography, or both, to any person who completes a state-approved course of training and passes an examination approved by the board.
Washington		Y	Y	The state also grants licensure to limited registered x-ray technicians. To obtain limited licensure, the student must pass the ARRT Limited Scope of Practice Examination after completing a state-approved course. The student must also attend an 8-hour HIV/AIDS training course at a local hospital or clinic prior to being granted licensure.
West Virginia		N		
Wisconsin	Y			
Wyoming		Y	Y	The state also grants restricted licensure. For restricted license status, a student must pass the ARRT Limited Scope of Practice in Radiography Examination with 80%.

Note: Alaska has no published guidelines.

TABLE 8.2
AHRA Staffing Ratio Survey Sample Table of Contents

(continued)

TABLE 8.2 (CONTINUED)
AHRA Staffing Ratio Survey Sample Table of Contents

Source: AHRA Staffing Ratio Survey (2006) Sample Table of Contents. With permission.

9 Policies and Procedures

Development of policies and procedures serves several purposes. First, it documents how things should be done or understood. It ensures consistency so there is no confusion.

Policies are more formal—typically representing rules. When policies are drafted, they should be understandable, clearly worded, and have the following components:

- Specific format
- Title
- Creation date
- Revision date
- Signoffs (administrator, department chair)

Procedures help to ensure consistency. They are used to implement policies. Procedures contain details on how to perform a task.

The main sections to develop are as follows:

- Department-Specific Mission/Vision
- Human Resources
- Administrative
- Financial
- Equipment
- File Room/Registration
- Picture Archiving and Communication System (PACS)
- Radiology Information System (RIS)
- Safety
- Radiation Protection
- Patient Care
- HIV, Isolation, Latex Allergy, etc.
- Documents (reports, orders, scheduling, etc.)
- Quality Control
- Modality Specific Procedures
- Facility Procedures
- Bomb Threat, Weather, etc.

This list is not comprehensive. Policies and procedures will depend on the type of institution, imaging procedures performed, and a variety of other factors.

A sample imaging policy and procedure manual can be found online at http://www.ahraonline.org/AM/Template.cfm?Section=Home&Template=/Search/SearchDisplay.cfm.

The following pages contain samples of policies, procedures, and some suggested topics.

Sample Policy

REGIONAL MEDICAL CENTER

POLICIES AND PROCEDURES: MEDICAL IMAGING SERVICES

Effective Date:	Reference No.:
Revised Date:	Category:
Reviewed by:	Director, Imaging Services
	Medical Director, Imaging Services

IMAGING SERVICES STAFF MEETINGS AND CONTINUING EDUCATION POLICY

1.0 Purpose: Staff in-services education shall be scheduled for all caregivers on a regular basis.

2.0 Procedure

- 2.1 Monthly staff meetings will be conducted at which protocol changes can be explained and discussed.
  - a) It is mandatory to attend or read the monthly staff meetings—caregivers must sign the monthly sign-in sheet. This will affect the caregiver's yearly evaluation.
  - b) The minutes will be posted in the radiology lounge for 2 months.
- 2.2 Yearly education requirements are to be completed for the annual and 90-day probations for all new caregivers in Imaging Services.
- 2.3 New equipment—mandatory in-service for all caregivers using the equipment.
- 2.4 CPR where required for the caregivers job.
- 2.5 Mandatory meeting set up by hospital and management for in-services.

3.0 Guidelines

- 3.1 Team leader in each department will check the outpatient schedule to verify the schedules are blocked.
  - a) If not blocked, please inform the radiology supervisor and/or designee.
- 3.2 CD, videos, or exam tested may be needed for in-services.
- 3.3 Attendance at national, state and local seminars will be based on staffing needs and granted as deemed appropriate by the imaging services director and/or radiology supervisor.

Policy prepared by:
Reviewed/Approved by: Imaging Department Director

Sample Procedure

Refer to Table 9.1.

Sample Table of Contents[1]

- Department Overview
- Hours of Operation/Staffing

TABLE 9.1
Sample Procedure

Regional Medical Center
Department of Radiology
Multidetector CT Protocols
GE Lightspeed +
L-Spine

Application:	Limited
Mode:	Helical
Kv/mAs/Time per rotation (sec):	120/250/1sec
Detector Collimation/Slice Thickness (mm):	4×1.25
Table speed (mm per rotation)/Pitch:	3.75/0.75:1
Data Reconstruction (mm):	1.25
Oral Contrast:	None
IV Contrast Type/Amount/Injection Rate:	None
Algorithim:	Standard
SFOV:	Large
FOV:	25.0cm adjust as needed
Scan Delay (sec):	None

Source: AHRA, Policies TOC. With permission.
Notes:

1. Scouts
   A. 0 & 90 degree from top of T12 through bottom of sacrum.
2. Helical Run
   A. 1.25mm slices from middle of vertebrae above area of interest to middle of vertebrae below area of interest. *(Do Not Angle)*
3. Reconstructions
   A. Do coronal and sagittal reformats of entire spine.
   B. Do 3-Ds in 360-degree rotation, top to bottom and left to right at radiologist's request.
4. PACS
   A. Send all images to QC1; include any reformats or 3-Ds.
5. Filming
   A. Film soft tissue windows.

- Radiologists
- Individual Department Plan
- Types of Service
- Ages of Patients Served
- Goals
- Scope of Services
- Care or Service Delivery Method
- Assignments
- Staffing Plan
- Verbal Orders

- Ordering Privileges
- Physician Orders
- Operation of Radiology Equipment
- Requesting Radiologic Exams
- Scheduling Outpatient Diagnostic Procedures
- Scheduling of Needle Localizations Prior to Surgery
- Scheduling of Patients with Known Latex Allergy
- Canceled Procedure Charting and Corporate Compliance
- Processing Patients during Planned Computer Downtime
- Informed Consent
- Consent for Invasive Procedures or Conscious Sedation
- Consent to Treatment/Informed Consent
- Guidelines for Radiology Usage in Other Areas

INTERVENTIONAL RADIOLOGY

- Patient Identification and Marking of Surgical Site
- Discharge Planning Assessment
- Procedures Standard
- History and Physicals (Requirements) Standard
- Post-Procedure Status
- Scope of Reassessment
- Standard

HUMAN RESOURCES

- Certification Requirements—Technologists
- Notification of Inability to Report for Duty
- Telephone Courtesy
- Clock-in/Clock-out Procedures
- Overtime
- X-Ray Room Care
- Evening Shift Technologists' Responsibilities/Duties
- Night Shift Technologist Duties
- Staff Meetings
- Tardiness and Fractional Overtime
- Safety
- Employee Safety Responsibility
- Internal Disaster
- Incident Report Form
- Patient/Visitor Property Loss or Damage
- Employee Incident Reporting
- Competency and Skill Verification Summary Sheet
- Job Description Addendum—Age Specific Criteria
- Confidentiality Statement
- Diagnostic X-Ray Department Orientation
- Age and Skill Competency Verification Sheet
- Venipuncture Policy

EQUIPMENT

- Equipment Management Plans
- Preventive Maintenance
- Electrical Safety
- Quality Control
- Medical Device Reporting
- (Alternative or Supplement to) Reporting Adverse Medical
- Expected Reporting Data Elements
- Imaging Equipment Purchase Evaluations
- Imaging Equipment Incoming Inspection
- Imaging Equipment Orientation, In-Service Training, and Competency
- Equipment Lock-Out, Tag-Out
- Monitoring Imaging Patient Care Equipment Vendors
- Parts Requisition System
- Product/Device Hazard Recalls
- Imaging Patient Care Equipment Repair/Replacement
- Radiological Engineering Safety
- Radiological Engineering Corrective Work Order System
- Technical Literature

FILM FILE MANAGEMENT

- Film Availability
- Copies
- Storage
- Report Turnaround Time
- Report for Incomplete Exam
- Films and Record Ownership and Patient Access

GENERAL SAFETY

- General Safety
- Safety Inspection Checklist
- Patient Handling/Care of the Back
- Electrical Hazard Prevention
- Evacuation Procedures
- Equipment Safety
- Mechanical Safety
- Environmental Management/Safety Plan
- Procedure for Response to a Fire
- Fire and Explosion
- Tornado Alert and Warning
- Bomb Threat
- Suspected Bomb Discovery
- Internal Disaster
- Incident Report Form
- Employee Incident Reporting
- Inpatient Incident
- Outpatient or Visitor Incident
- Patient/Visitor Property Loss or Damage

- Violent Situation Alert
- Workplace Violence Prevention Plan
- Employee Contact with Hazardous Materials
- Handling and Disposal of Hazardous Materials
- Hazardous Material Program
- Employee Safety Responsibility
- Sentinel Event

INFECTION CONTROL

- General Policy Statements
- Environmental Considerations
- Supplies and Accessories
- Traffic Control for Imaging Procedures
- Portable Equipment— Disinfectant Cleaning
- Standard Infection Control Precautions Policies
- Personnel Responsibilities
- Biohazardous Materials: Needles and Other Sharps
- Isolation Attire
- Portable Exams for Patients Requiring Contact, Droplet, or Airborne Precautions
- Standard Precautions: Soiled/Used Linens
- Waste Management Precautions: Waste Disposal
- Disposal of Body Waste
- Ultrasound "Endo" Transducer Disinfection Process "CIDEX OPA"

PATIENT CARE

- Preps for Special Radiologic Procedures
- Pediatric Preps for Diagnostic Procedures
- Patient Information and Preparations
- Prep Procedure for CT Scans
- Appropriateness Indications Disclaimer
- Clinical Indications for Exam
- Exam Appropriateness and Screening
- General Policies Regarding Privacy, Contrast Media, and Removal for Patient Care
- Patient Responsibilities
- Patient Rights
- Patient Rights to Consent/Refusal for Treatment
- Care/Handling for Suspected Spinal Fracture Patients
- Patient Safety
- Transportation—Requisition Information
- Transportation Information and Procedure—General
- Transportation Policy—Mode of Transport
- Transportation—Sign Out Procedure
- Transportation of Patients with IVs
- Transportation Policy—Infants
- Transportation Policy—Isolation Patients
- Transportation of Critically Ill Patient
- Critical Care Transport

- Care and Handling of Critically Ill Patients
- Use of/Changing IV Solutions
- Medications in Radiology
- Contrast Reaction Policy
- IV Contrast Administration Procedure
- Treatment of Reaction to Contrast Media
- (CPR # 1) Cardiac/Respiratory Arrest
- (CPR #2) Code 99/Cardiopulmonary Resuscitation
- Nursing Observation Area—Radiology
- Employees' Responsibility Regarding Latex Sensitivity
- Alert Systems for Latex Sensitive Patients
- Products to Be Used for Latex-Sensitive Patients
- Room Preparation for Latex-Sensitive Patients
- Contents of Latex-Sensitivity Kit and Location
- Magnetic Exposure
- Urinary Catheterization
- Conscious Sedation
- Adverse Drug Reaction Reporting
- Medication Errors
- Iodinated Contrast Agent Selection
- MRI Safety/Screening
- Ostomy Pouching
- Suctioning, Oropharyngeal, and Nasopharyngeal
- Pulse Oximetry
- Unsealed Sources
- Advance Directives
- Patient Rights to Care and Comfort
- Patient Rights and Responsibilities
- Patients with History of Allergies or Contraindications

RADIATION SAFETY

- Radiation/Fluoroscopy Safety
- Noninterpretive Fluoroscopy
- Prenatal Radiation Exposure
- Instructions Concerning Pregnant Employees
- Radiation Safety Committee
- Medical Radiation Physicist Responsibilities (Option 1)
- Medical Radiation Physicist Responsibilities (Option 2)
- ALARA Program
- General Rules of Radiation Safety
- Repeat Exams
- Persons Permitted in X-Ray Rooms
- Radiation Safety Rules for Portable Radiography
- Patients Receiving Therapeutic Radioactive Materials

NUCLEAR MEDICINE

- Nuclear Medicine Equipment Quality Control Schedule
- Survey Instrument Calibration
- Radioactive Waste Management

- Written Directive for Radiopharmaceuticals
- Procurement, Storage, Distribution, and Preparation of Medication Dose System for Radiopharmaceuticals
- Administration of Radiopharmaceuticals in Nuclear Medicine
- Wipe Tests and Area Surveys
- Handling of Radioactive Sealed Sources
- Radiation Safety Checklist for Iodine Therapy over 30 mCi
- I Therapy Room Survey Report
- Administration of Radioactive Iodine Dose > 30 mCi
- Record for the Administration of Radioiodine > 30 mCi
- 131-I Thyroid Therapy Checklist

RESULTS REPORTING

- General Guidelines
- Addenda/Corrected Reports

MAGNETIC RESONANCE IMAGING

- Restricted Magnetic Field Area Defined
- Caution in Handling Objects Near Magnetic Field
- Claustrophobia and Sedation
- Patient Pregnancy
- Fetal MRI Examination
- Personnel and Visitor Screening
- Response to a Fire
- Safe Handling of Liquid Helium and Liquid Nitrogen
- Precautions for Emergency Equipment
- Electrical Safety
- Magnet Safety
- Cryogen Safety
- Preventive Maintenance of MRI Scanner
- Housekeeping
- Employee Pregnancy
- Hazard/Warning Communication
- Procedure for Response to Low Oxygen Alarm
- Magnet Quench
- Removal of Magnetic Field
- Restarting the Superconductive Magnet
- Scanning Protocols
- Call Policy for Emergency Scans
- Patient Information and Preparations
- Patient Screening
- Patient Questionnaire
- Outside Referrals
- Devices Safely Scanned with MRI 1 5 Tesla
- Contraindications to MRI Scanning
- Warning of MRI Scanning and Effects

MAMMOGRAPHY

- Interpreting Physicians' Qualifications
- Technologists' Qualification Requirements
- Mammography Technologists' Orientation
- Technologists' Performance Requirements
- Technologists' Restrictions
- Physicists' Qualifications
- Physicists' Responsibilities
- Personnel Records Retention
- Mammography Services
- Patient Selection Criteria
- Scheduling Mammography Patients
- Comparison of Previous Films
- Exam Preparation
- Screening Mammography Standing Orders
- Diagnostic Mammography
- Breast Implant Imaging
- Mammographic Image Identification
- Repeat Film
- Mammography Patients' Notification of Results
- Follow-Up for Abnormal Mammography Results
- Self-Referred Patients
- Mammography Tracking
- Mammography Film Retention and Release
- Mammography Quality Assurance Program
- Mammography Assurance Responsibility
- Equipment Quality Control
- Quality Control Test Results
- Department Cleanliness
- Infection Control
- Quality Assurance Records
- Patient Complaints
- Mammography Medical Outcomes Audit

REFERENCE

1. Courtesy of the American Healthcare Radiology Administrators, www.ahraonline.org

10 Conducting Meetings and Facilitating

CONDUCTING MEETINGS

Conducting and overseeing meetings is a very important skill. It represents a repeatable, organized way to disseminate information, brainstorm, and solicit involvement and buy-in (Image 10.1).

The first step in meeting organization is to define the type of meeting. Will it be held to distribute general informational, to focus on a specific topic, to solicit feedback, or something else?

Steps to conducting a meeting:

a. Solicit topic input
b. Develop agenda
c. Distribute agenda, request feedback
d. Manage attendees

One of the hardest tasks in conducting meetings is to keep attendees on task. To accomplish this, it is important that the start time be firm. It is very disruptive to have people wandering in after the meeting has begun. Make sure there are no side discussions going on between attendees. Keep on topic and task. Limit time for any one participant—this reduces "meandering diatribe."

Keeping effective minutes means documenting all of the important aspects and topics covered. Remember, meeting minutes can be used for legal purposes, so be careful of what is contained in them. It is not necessary to record every word or conversation held. It will suffice to state "discussion ensued" or some such wording to record the fact that interchange did take place. Other elements that should be contained are the title, date and time, a listing of attendees and absentees, and decisions/conclusions. Also assign follow-up topics and deadlines and document these.

Distribute minutes soon after the meeting, while your memory is still fresh. Make sure there are backup copies somewhere. Many times you will have to refer to past meeting minutes to clarify an issue (Image 10.2).

FACILITATING

Facilitating is different from leading a meeting. Facilitating is typically used for brainstorming-type sessions. The facilitator is also an *enabler,* eliciting feedback from attendees. She or he could also be thought of as more of a "ringleader" than a meeting leader. A major role of the facilitator is to keep the fact-finding or decision-making process moving.

The facilitator should distribute comments ahead of the meeting to spark ideas and opinions that can be brought to the session. After a general overview of the topic or topics at hand, the attendees should be split into smaller workgroups. The facilitator should then assign topics or goals for each workgroup. This helps to move processes along.

Toward the end of the session, a group spokesman should present the group's ideas or data. The facilitator should then determine how the data will be presented. The facilitator should also be nonjudgmental as much as prudently possible.

There are many different ways to build consensus, explore facts, and make decisions. The topic will determine which method is best for working with it.

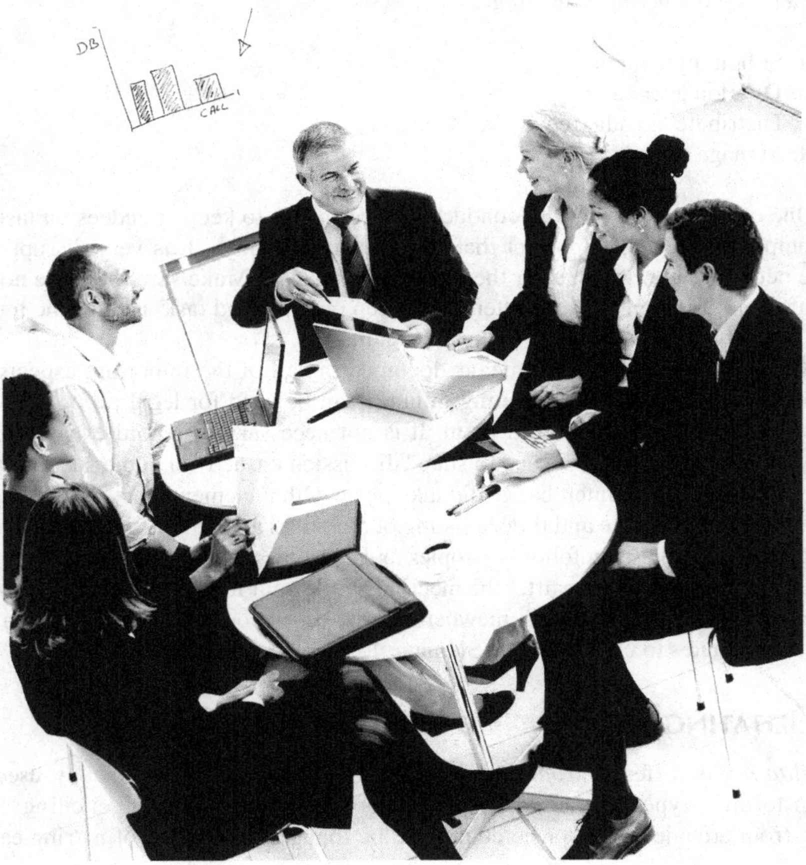

IMAGE 10.1 Meeting facilitation is an important skill.

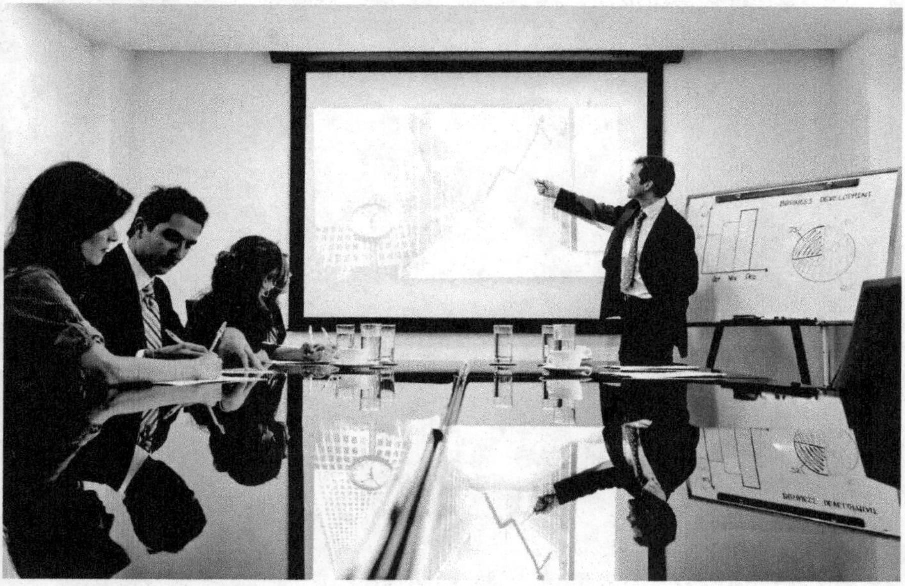

IMAGE 10.2

11 PACS/RIS Workflow

PACS—picture archiving and communication system—has replaced conventional film and film jackets for storage, retrieval, and archiving of imaging studies.

RIS is an acronym for radiology information system, which is software specifically designed for the needs of an imaging department. It typically interfaces with the institution HIS, which stands for hospital information system, which integrates all clinical and business software. Integrated with the HIS, PACS handles data associated with images and RIS deals with financial, patient, and other information. This information is retrieved from and passed to the HIS.

Planning for PACS and RIS is a huge undertaking. In many cases it is the first attempt to transition from a paper to a computerized system.

The first advice is do not try to be an expert. PACS and RIS administrators are specially trained for the more technical aspects of PACS and RIS. Outside consultants can also be utilized.

It is important to get radiologists involved from the beginning. At that point, the manager should determine an evaluation team and determine available resources from staff (experience, etc.). If needed, involve a consultant. The consultant does not have to be used for the entire project.

Others who should be on the team include:

1. Radiology administrator
2. PACS/RIS administrator
3. Radiologist champion
4. Medical staff/physician champion
5. Facility IT
6. Facility financial person
7. File room supervisor
8. Nursing
9. Radiology staff

THE PRE-INSTALL PHASE

Obviously much planning must go into a PACS/RIS project before the installation can begin. One of the documents resulting is called a *request for proposal*, or RFP, which is a long list of detailed questions as to how the vendor's product will meet the needs of the requestor. PACS/RIS vendors can assist with the workflow and design considerations so that you ask the right questions in the RFP. The RFP should contain a deadline date and include all costs involved. Costs include warranty coverage and period, and what service contracts or pay-per-incident costs will be. Another important request is for guaranteed uptime. In most situations, this will be for a 24/7 scenario. In addition, there will be costs for interfaces. PACS/RIS/HIS vendors may not mention these, so it is important to ask about them!

An important component of the request is training, which should be part of the purchase package and should include what will be covered, where the training will take place, who should attend, who should become *superusers* (those caregivers in the institution who will be high-level users and possibly trainers). Inquire about what kind of expenses might be incurred for travel and lodging for training.

When researching PACS and RIS, use resources such as MD Buyline, a company that researches products and vendors for a fee and returns the results to the institution. Investigate online resources—vendor websites and others.

The next step in the process is to analyze, document, and chart processes. This includes where devices will be kept, how they will be used and by whom, and how traffic—both electronic and people traffic—will flow.

When planning the install process, set goals with dates and be sure to leave "slush" room. Unexpected delays will almost always occur.

Learn PACS/RIS lingo. It is a language of its own, and the ability to understand the terms used is vital. Again vendors can help here.

Which modalities will be connected? X-ray, CT, ultrasound, and others? For each of these modalities an interface will be necessary to pass data to and from the modality. The interface will result in higher costs.

Quality control considerations need to be made. Look at what the vendor offers as far as the ability to review and change images and their associated data. Keying errors occur in daily use, as well as incorrect demographic information associating with the wrong images. There are other issues that come up regularly, so look for a product that has considered these possibilities and done as much possible to prevent them. Processes involving the QC (quality control) of workstations also must be put in place.

Of extreme importance are *security and HIPAA (patient privacy) considerations*. Ask the vendor what precautions are in place to ensure restricted access and security of patient data.

Backup and redundancy of data used by PACS/RIS is vital. At minimum, daily backups of patient data should be made, preferably to an offsite storage location.

There are also considerations when choosing or changing a PACS/RIS. There is a need to have the vendors under consideration explain the "upgrade path." This spells out future software upgrades—how they are handled, what the functionality changes will be, training needs, and costs. Also inquire about hardware upgrade costs.

DICOM considerations must also be made. DICOM is a standard for digital image processing. It is a must that DICOM format be handled by the RIS/PACS and HIS (hospital) in order to pass information among them in a systematic, accurate fashion.

If the department is going from a film-based system or changing to a different vendor's PACS/RIS, a transition plan of how this will be accomplished must be done. In most cases the vendors will have all of these considerations and details outlined for the end users. Among these is the transition of the film library—getting film images into a digital format. Prior studies must be available. Some institutions will keep prior film-based studies on hand and over time prior film studies can be disposed of. Other institutions will scan films. Scanning is a very expensive and tedious process. Most institutions will scan prior film studies as needed.

The importance of the PACS/RIS/HIS *integration* cannot be emphasized enough. Vendors of the various components must ensure their product will integrate seamlessly with others. Make sure to get this guarantee in writing! Also be mindful that the institutions will have to purchase separate interfaces between these components. Make sure these are included in the vendor quotes.

Ensure that proper training is done. Vendors will have applications specialists that will train end users. Some train a few key personnel, known as *superusers*, who will then train the remainder of the staff, depending on their job responsibilities.

When training, it is important to ask, "Who will be adding information to the system?"

Here is a short list:

- Input clerks/registration
- Technologists
- Radiologists
- Offsite scheduling
- Others

The next questions to ask are, "Who will be using the information?" and "What information will be included?" Voice recognition technology should be considered.

- Radiologists
- Referring physician offices
- Preps
- Exam information
- ER
- OR
- Management for reporting
- Billing
- Risk management
- Others

Some of the major advantages of moving to a PACS/RIS:

- Faster access to reports and studies
- Virtually no loss of documents/studies
- Access by many at the same time
- Storage—long and short term

A radiologist "champion" should be chosen. Some of the radiologist workflow considerations are as follows:

- Onsite locations
- Ambient lighting, noise

- Teleradiology reading areas
- QC technologist interactions
- Staff technologists interactions
- File room personnel interactions
- Studies sent to or from offsite facilities
- View boxes for nondigitized studies
- Ability and ease of reading studies
- Availability of offsite reading

There are consultants who specialize in the entire PACS/RIS project. Peers should also be consulted.

12 Quality

Quality in medical imaging is wide in terms of scope. The two main aspects to quality considerations in imaging management are management quality and technical quality.

Quality management is an ongoing evaluation of clinical equipment and processes.
Continuous quality improvement (CQI) is an ongoing evaluation of processes affecting outcomes.

A background of quality management is helpful in understanding what tools are available for the imaging manager.

W. Edwards Deming focused on the use of statistical quality control.
Joseph M. Juran focused on managing for quality.
Walter A. Shewhart is known as the "father of statistical control."
Total quality management, also known as TQM, is a broad business concept that includes the CQI process.

Some other terms are as follows:

- CQI
- Process improvement (PI)
- Plan, Do, Check, Act (PDCA)
- 85/15 Rule
- Six Sigma
- Lean

The 85/15 rule states, "When something goes wrong, 85% of the problem is related to systems failure; 15% is the fault of the people involved" (W. Edwards Deming).

SIX SIGMA

- Six Sigma seeks to identify and remove the causes of defects and errors in manufacturing and business processes.
- Six Sigma means that over the long-term, a process will produce fewer than 3.5 defects per million opportunities.
- A defect is anything that could lead to customer dissatisfaction.
- It is very data driven and not an appropriate improvement method for everything.
- This is a rigorous process, and staff need to be specially challenged to lead Six Sigma initiatives.

LEAN

Lean is increasing customer value by eliminating waste throughout the value stream.

The Seven Wastes in Healthcare

1. Defects: Resticks, med errors, repeating tests, missing charts, lost test results
2. Overproduction: Producing "just-in-case" IV solutions without orders, blood drawn early to accommodate the lab
3. Inventories: Patients waiting for bed assignments, lab samples with batched dictation waiting for transcription, excess supplies, x-rays stacked in an in-box
4. Movement: Looking for patients, missing meds, missing charts or equipment
5. Extra Processing: Multiple bed moves, retesting, multiple approvals, auditing
6. Transportation: Moving patients to tests, moving materials, moving patients in and out of rooms
7. Waiting: Inpatients waiting in the emergency department, patients waiting for discharge, patients waiting to be seen, physicians waiting for test results or charts

DEMING'S 14 POINTS

Deming's 14 points are principles for management for transforming the effectiveness of a business. Deming's work was done mainly in the nonmedical side of business. However, his principles have been adapted.

1. Create constancy of purpose to improve service. Aim to be competitive, stay in business, and provide jobs.
2. Adopt a new philosophy.
3. Cease dependence on mass inspection for quality.
4. Build quality into the product from the beginning.
5. Do not award business on price alone.
6. Minimize cost and use JIT (just in time, also called Kanban). JIT is a type of inventory control that orders only what is immediately needed, with no stockpiling of supplies.
7. Continually improve service.
8. Institute on-the-job training, education, and self-improvement programs.
9. Provide leadership to help people do their jobs better.
10. Drive out fear.
11. Break down departmental barriers.
12. Eliminate slogans and targets.
13. Eliminate merit rating systems.
14. Involve the entire organization in total quality improvement.

SURVEYS

Surveys are tools that can be used to assess quality in imaging. They can be used for direct patient input, as well as referring physician and staff input. The information can be used for determining levels of customer satisfaction and for marketing purposes.

The most common surveys in medical imaging are as follows:

- Patient satisfaction surveys
- Referring physician surveys
- Staff satisfaction surveys

Survey Instrument Considerations

- Survey design should generate actionable and valid data—need to write good questions
- Use a interval scale such as the Likert scale
- Statistical confidence
- Response rates
- Reduce bias
- Data input
- Data analysis
- Cover letters
- Pilots

Types of Survey Questions

- Multiple choice
- Ordinal
- Interval
- Ratio
- Open-ended text

Survey Questions

- Surveys should be as short as possible.
- Questions should be simple and unambiguous.
- Preprinted answers that can be ticked are best.
- Questions should be relevant and not too personal.
- Questions should fall into a logical sequence.
- Avoid leading questions.

STATISTICAL TOOLS

A variety of statistical tools are available for the imaging manager to use. The use will depend on what is to be accomplished or studied.

Histograms show frequency distribution (how often something occurs). See Graph 12.1.

Fishbone diagrams which are a representation of possible cause of a problem. See Graphic 12.1.

Run charts have upper and lower control limits. In Graph 12.2, the upper and lower limits, designated by the straight lines, could represent minimum and maximum body temperatures that are being monitored over a time period. You can see that if the data points are above or below the control limits, some type of action should be taken.

MEDICAL INDUSTRY REGULATIONS

Medicine is a very highly regulated industry. Healthcare is a heavily regulated industry subject to a myriad and sometimes complex sets of rules governing coverage and reimbursement of medical services. Noncompliance with federal- and state-sponsored healthcare programs presents substantial risks to the healthcare provider. Government agencies can recoup improper payment and impose sanctions. This applies to *all* entities receiving payments for Medicare and Medicaid services. The program is called Corporate Compliance Initiative (CCI) and must contain the following elements:

- Development and distribution of policies, procedures, and standards of conduct
- The appointment of a chief compliance officer
- An education and training program
- A process for complaints
- A response system for allegations
- Procedures for audits and evaluations
- Investigation and mediation of any problems

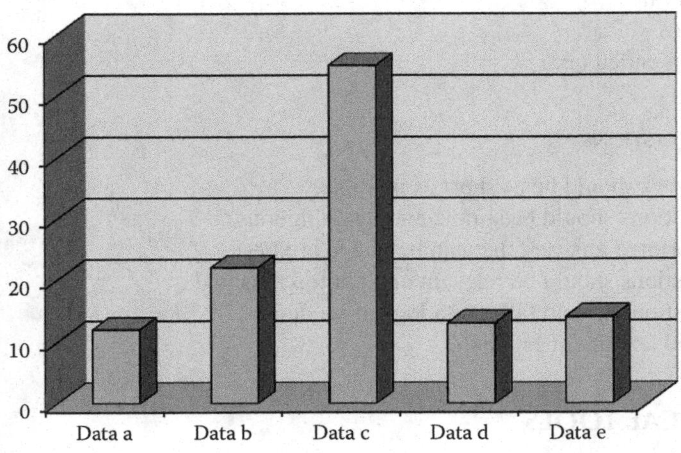

GRAPH 12.1 Bar chart.

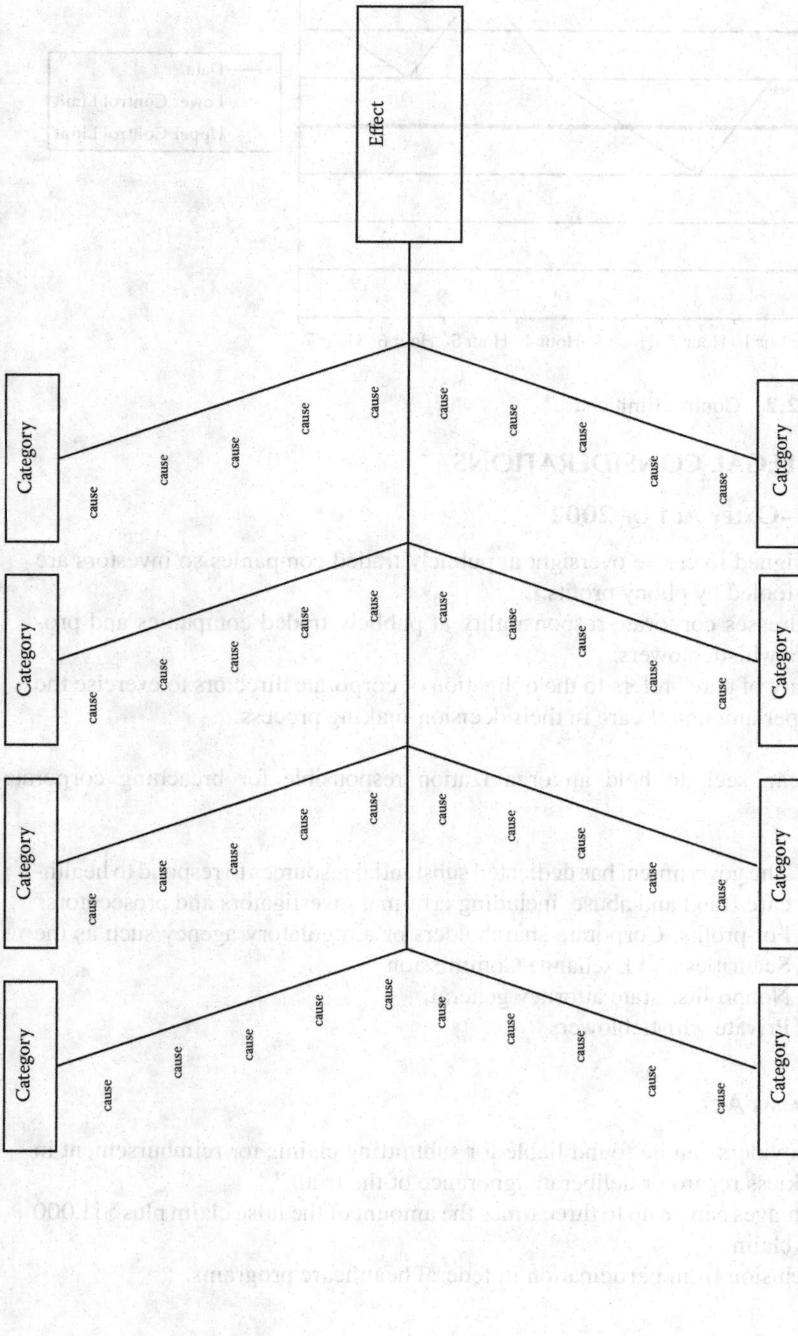

GRAPHIC 12.1 Fishbone diagram.

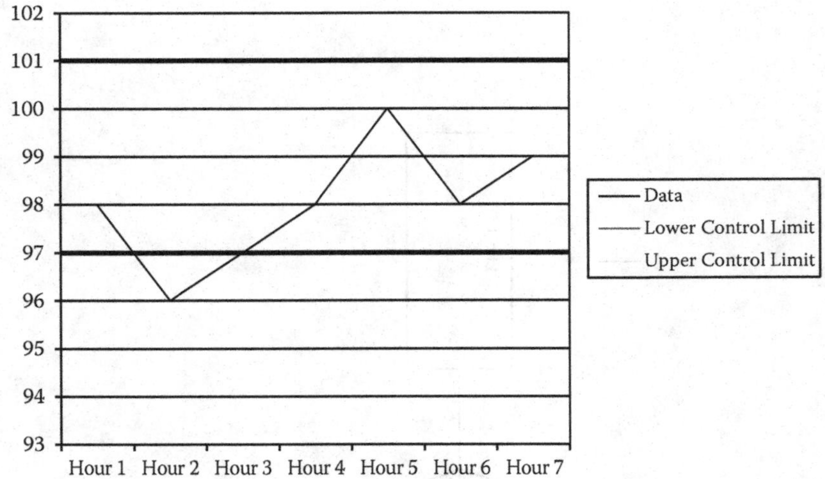

GRAPH 12.2 Control limit chart.

OTHER LEGAL CONSIDERATIONS

Sarbanes–Oxley Act of 2002

- Designed to create oversight at publicly traded companies so investors are not fooled by phony profits.
- Addresses corporate responsibility at publicly traded companies and protects whistleblowers.
- "Duty of care" refers to the obligation of corporate directors to exercise the proper amount of care in their decision-making process.

Who can seek to hold an organization responsible for breaching corporate compliance?

1. The government has dedicated substantial resources to respond to healthcare fraud and abuse, including criminal investigators and prosecutors.
2. For-profits: Corporate shareholders or a regulatory agency such as the Securities and Exchange Commission
3. Nonprofits: State attorney general
4. Private whistleblowers

False Claims Act

- "Providers can be found liable for submitting claims for reimbursement in reckless regard or deliberate ignorance of the truth."
- Damages can be up to three times the amount of the false claim plus $11,000 per claim.
- Exclusion from participation in federal healthcare programs.

Types of Medicare Fraud

- "Phantom billing"—billing for tests not performed
- Performing inappropriate or unnecessary procedures
- Charging for supplies/equipment never ordered
- Billing for new equipment when old equipment was used
- Billing for expensive equipment when nonexpensive equipment was used
- "Reflex testing"—automatically performing a test whenever the results of some other test fall within a certain range, even though the reflex test was not ordered by a physician
- Defective testing—billing for a test that was not or only partially performed because of technical difficulties
- "Code jamming"—laboratories inserting or "jamming" fake diagnosis codes to get Medicare/Medicaid coverage
- "Unbundling"—using 2 or more CPT billing codes instead of one inclusive code for a defined panel where rules and regulations require "bundling" of such claims
- Submitting multiple bills to obtain a higher reimbursement for tests and services that were performed within a specified time period and that should have been submitted as a single bill
- Double billing—charging more than once for the same service
- Upcoding—inflating bills by using dx (diagnostic) codes that indicate the patient experienced medical complications or needed more expensive treatments, billing for complex services when only simple services were performed, billing for brand-name drugs when generic drugs were provided
- "Phantom employees"—expensing employees or hours worked that do not exist
- Improper cost reports—submitting false cost reports seeking Medicare reimbursements higher than permitted by actual facts
- Providing substandard nursing home care and seeking Medicare reimbursement
- Routinely waiving patient copayments

FBI Arrests Hospital Executives for Medicare Fraud

The *New York Sun* reported on August 8, 2008, that hospitals in Los Angeles and Orange counties used homeless people, drug addicts, and the mentally ill as "human pawns." These "patients" were picked by recruiters who sent them to a skid row health assessment center. There they were given a phony diagnosis and forms were filled out justifying their eligibility for government medical programs. Medicare and Medi-Cal would be billed for the ambulance and hospital stay. After their hospital stay, the "patients" were returned to skid row shelters. "Patients were paid $20–$30 for each hospital stay. The recruiters received $40 for each Medicare patient and $20 for each Medi-Cal patient. The three hospitals that were involved in the scheme billed Medicare and Medi-Cal for millions of dollars."

Kennedy–Kassenbaum Bill

Also known as the Health Insurance Portability and Accountability Act of 1996 (HIPAA), the intent of the Kennedy–Kassenbaum bill was to eliminate preexisting condition clauses that prevented Americans from retaining or acquiring health insurance when they changed jobs or moved to another state. Under the authority of HIPAA, the Department of Health and Human Services has written guidelines for the protection and privacy of a patient's healthcare records. All providers of healthcare services must comply with HIPAA guidelines. The legislation extends limits to private insurance companies as well as Medicare.

Stark Law

The Stark Law is named for Congressman Pete Stark who sponsored the initial bill. This legislation governs physician self-referral. Self-referral is the practice of referring a patient to a medical facility in which he/she has a financial interest.

The Stark law was initiated to prevent "kickback" arrangements. It prohibits physicians from referring business to an entity in which they have a financial interest. It also prohibits giving discretionary discounts, including courtesy discounts or write-offs that were historically given to physicians and their families. Violators can be punished by not being allowed to participate in Medicare, charged fines, or even imprisoned.

Mammography Quality Standards Act

The Mammography Quality Standards Act (MQSA) mandates that sites be accredited in order to receive Medicare funding. MQSA was the only federal quality and safety standards in place prior to July 9, 2008.

MQSA accepts accreditation by the American College of Radiology (ACR). ACR accreditation ensures that physicians supervising and interpreting medical imaging meet stringent education and training standards, imaging equipment is surveyed regularly by qualified medical physicists to ensure that it is functioning properly, and technologists administering the tests are appropriately certified.

Another accepted accrediting agency is the Intersocietal Accreditation Commission (IAC).

Many payers and insurance companies have adapted MQSA and require that sites be certified. Below is a sample list of payers that require accreditation:

- Blue Cross Blue Shield of Kansas City
- Anthem Blue Cross Blue Shield Indiana, Kentucky, Ohio
- United Healthcare (will accept ACR or IAC)
- Anthem Health Plans of Virginia
- Aetna

Some payers require that other modalities, such as nuclear medicine, be certified by an accrediting agency. There are several agencies besides the ACR that are accepted. Below is a sample list of payers that require nuclear medicine accreditation:

- Anthem Health Plans of Virginia
- United Healthcare Wisconsin
- Anthem Blue Cross Blue Shield Indiana, Kentucky, Ohio
- Highmark Blue Cross Blue Shield Pennsylvania
- Care Core National
- Oxford Health Plan Connecticut

CMS (Centers for Medicare and Medicaid Services) Accreditation Requirements

The Medicare Improvements for Patients and Providers Act of 2008 (MIPPA) requires providers of imaging services to be accredited by January 1, 2012. Accreditation is mandatory for payment for the technical component of imaging services. The *technical component* is the part paid to the hospital or imaging center. The *professional component* is that paid to the radiologist. These will be explained in more detail in Chapter 14.

United Healthcare Imaging Accreditation Program

United Healthcare, or UHC, is one of the largest payers in the country. UHC requires outpatient imaging sites and providers that bill on a CMS/HICF 1500 or its electronic equivalent (this is a form used for Medicare) and perform CT, MR, PET, nuclear medicine, nuclear cardiology, and echocardiography to be accredited. Accreditation applies to global and technical service claims. (Global billing will be explained in Chapter 14.)

ACR Accreditations

- Mammography
- Radiation Oncology
- Breast Ultrasound
- CT
- MR
- Nuclear Medicine and PET
- Ultrasound
- Stereotactic Breast Biopsy
- Breast Imaging Center of Excellence

Organizations and Acts

AAAHC—Association for the Accreditation of Ambulatory Healthcare Facilities
ACHE—American College of Healthcare Executives (www.ache.org)
ACR—American College of Radiology (www.acr.org)
AHRA—American Healthcare Radiology Administrators (www ahraonline.org)
ARRT—American Registry of Radiologic Technologists (www.arrt.org)
CMS—Centers for Medicare and Medicaid Services
HIPAA—Health Insurance Portability and Accountability Act of 1996 (Kennedy–Kassenbaum Bill)
MIPPA—Medicare Improvements for Patients and Providers Act of 2008

TECHNICAL QUALITY

The quality of imaging devices must be maintained and tested on a regular basis. Quality control in imaging is the ongoing measurement and evaluation of clinical equipment and processes. A medical physicist should be used to set specifications and monitor them on an ongoing basis for accreditation and quality. Physical quality control consists of radiation protection, x-ray beam characteristics, screen-film characteristics, digital imaging systems, and in some cases, conventional film processing.

COLLECTION AND ANALYSIS OF QUALITY CONTROL DATA

The following tests should be run on a regular basis, according to manufacturer specifications:

- Generator performance
- Beam characteristics
- Ancillary equipment evaluations
- Fluoroscopic systems
- Processor performance
- Imaging system performance
- Evaluation of digital systems

Test Instrumentation

- kVp evaluation
- Radiation detector
- Length of exposure
- Test objects, phantoms
- Sensitometer
- Densitometer
- Light meter
- Test pattern generator

There is a wide spectrum of testing that must be done on a regular basis. It is best to contact a medical physicist to fill in the details.

Other Quality Control Data

There are other areas of imaging that should be monitored. A few suggestions are as follows:

Radiology/Pathology correlation—When a biopsy is done in the imaging department, the pathology report should be obtained so that the radiologist can confirm his or her diagnosis.

Repeat Rate—The number of repeats by technologist should be monitored. At a minimum, data collected should state the reason for the repeat, the view repeated, and the body part. This should be used as a coaching tool for technologists on a regular basis. The national average for repeat rate (without students) is 3 to 5%.

Radiologist Peer Review—A sampling of cases should be over-read by a different radiologist than the one who originally read the case. This acts as a "check and balance" system for the radiologists to ensure that nothing is missed.

CT for Pulmonary Embolism—It is required by CMS at the writing of this book that all positive findings in CT for pulmonary embolism be followed up immediately with the ordering physician. This requires the radiologist to contact the ordering physician as soon as possible to discuss the case. The case information and the conversation should be documented.

Teleradiology Monitoring—If the radiologist group is using a teleradiology service for after-hours reads, sample cases should be reviewed by an in-house radiologist on a regular basis. This will ensure the quality of the reads.

Report Turnaround—Service quality in imaging is measured by two main factors: appointment accessibility and report turnaround. The time between the performance of the exam and when the report is actually communicated (by mail, fax, or e-mail) should be monitored on a regular basis. With the advent of digital imaging and voice recognition technologies, report turnaround has decreased from days to hours.

Emergency Room/Imaging Correlation—When an imaging exam is ordered by the emergency room, the images are typically viewed by the ER physician and initial treatment is based on that interpretation. The ER physician should note findings so that when the study is later read by a radiologist, the radiologist can contact the ER physician with any discrepancies. Many legal cases are based on lack of this type of "audit trail," so it is vital that this system be put into place.

There are a variety of quality parameters in addition to these that should be collected, analyzed, and reported upon, depending on institutional requirements and protocols.

13 Business Planning Basics

Business planning is a necessary part of today's healthcare. Reimbursement cuts continue, and expenses continue to rise.

Imaging departments and facilities are viewed as business units, whether located in a hospital or as part of an outpatient center. In many cases imaging profits help to bolster other revenue-negative departments or units.

The main components of a business plan are background, marketing, finance, goal formation, implementation and monitoring, and follow-up.

BACKGROUND

The background document is formulated to explain how and why the business unit exists and the history of the business unit, if any. It is also used to delineate the unique competencies. It is considered a "state of the department" (facility, etc.). This section of the business gives the general overall view of the business (department, imaging center, etc.).

MARKETING

Detailed information on marketing will be presented in Chapter 16. This section explains how marketing fits in the overall business plan.

To begin with, the mission/vision statement should drive marketing. It helps to explain the *why* of the business. In this portion of the plan, specific competencies are derived and explained—with statements such as "state-of-the-art mammography services." A service statement is then constructed, which describes how the business intends to meet and exceed demands and challenges.

The document should define business objectives in the short and long term—such as, meet and exceed monthly budget, add x new service lines by the end of the fiscal year. An industry description should be included, which defines trends, a general overview of the business segment, and other background material.

The target markets need to be defined. Is the business going after women, the elderly, others? Knowing target markets will help to narrow the focus during the marketing efforts.

An *environmental scan* should be performed to see what competitors are doing. This should include a SWOT analysis. This acronym stands for strengths, weaknesses, opportunities, and threats:

Strengths—what are the strengths of you facility of department? For example, cardiac imaging, women's services.
Weaknesses—for example, not enough after-hours availability.

Opportunities—Underserved markets, new procedures such as bone densitometry when Fosomax came out.
Threats
Internal—cardiologists, others doing exam volumes
External—imaging centers, local competitors

Next, the pricing levels for services should be determined or changed.

After this background work has been completed, promotional campaigns should be planned, along with sales and advertising plans. Last, a tracking or follow-up mechanism is developed. This will help to see what is working well and what is not, which can be followed by improvements and enhancements.

FINANCE

Budgets should be formulated to determine how much income and expense is expected. Various scenarios can be analyzed. Both operating and capital budgets should be constructed. The budget will help to determine what the profit will be after income is generated and expenses are paid.

The *variance analysis* is an ongoing, working document that tracks actual versus budgeted funds and volumes. It tracks where variance is—volume variance cause or cost variance.

Standard *financial statements* should be produced on a monthly basis. These statements follow FASB (Financial Accounting Standards Board) standards. They consist of internal and external documents.

The *statement of cash flows* is a standard financial report that answers the question: "Is there enough cash to coming in to cover current expenses?"

The *balance sheet* is a financial statement that states assets (what is owned) and liabilities (what is owed).

The *income statement* is generated, which denotes profit or loss for a given period.

GOAL FORMATION

The next part of the business plan is formation of goals. These must be achievable and realistic for your market. While forming goals, set target dates and financial constraints. Some examples of goals are as follows:

- More office hours
- Perform more procedures and/or new procedures
- Add equipment
- More equipment by modality
- New or replacement equipment
- Infrastructure (PACS, RIS, etc.)
- Increase service lines (add mammography, breast MRI, etc.)

IMPLEMENTATION AND ASSESSMENT

Monitoring or progress should occur over time including a periodic snapshot of where the plan is versus where it should be. This allows the team to make adjustments to improve performance and direction.

Keep informed of new technologies and procedures on the forefront and consider them if feasible and part of the plan.

Budget projections should be formulated and adjusted. The following items must be considered:

- Past volumes adjusted for changes in market
- Referring physician changes
- Staff radiologist changes
- Patient demographic changes
- New/expiring technology changes
- Legislative and regulatory changes
- Pricing changes
- Market changes in payer mix

A sample business plan for bone densitometry follows.

SAMPLE BUSINESS PLAN FOR BONE DENSITOMETRY

DESCRIPTION

Bone (mineral) density studies are used to evaluate diseases of bone and/or the responses of bone diseases to treatment. The studies assess bone mass or density associated with such diseases as osteoporosis, osteomalacia, and renal osteodystrophy. Various single or combined methods of measurement may be required to—

1. diagnose bone disease,
2. monitor the course of bone changes with disease progression, or
3. monitor the course of bone changes with therapy.

Bone density is usually studied by using photodensitometry, single- or dual-photon absorptiometry, or bone biopsy. Recent developments of pharmaceutical agents for treatment have elevated bone densitometry in the public awareness (see below under "Opportunities").

BUSINESS OBJECTIVES

- To provide bone densitometry studies to referring physicians at the clinic
- To be competitive in the bone densitometry market

- To provide possible spin-off referrals
- To continue to support women's services by offering bone densitometry in conjunction with mammography

MARKET/COMPETITIVE EVALUATION

Bone densitometry is not offered in the immediate area of the clinic. This service is offered at a nearby hospital.

RESOURCE COMMITMENT

Several vendors offer bone densitometry units. XYZ is one of the leaders in the product, and has offered a unit for $____.

A small room with one wall a minimum 9 feet in length is required. Other common area costs would be allocated.

The technologist for this procedure has an average salary of $____/hour.

CONSTRAINTS, RISKS

Demand for this technology is about at present is 6 to 10 cases/week. These requests appear to be independent of the hospital market.

Risk is involved in not offering this technology at the clinic. Due to the size, low cost, and low restrictions on installation, small offices and another nearby clinic may become market leaders in the immediate geographic area.

OPPORTUNITIES

There has been an increasing public awareness for this service. In addition, requests from referring physicians and the general public have been made at the clinic. This service could be offered in conjunction with other women's services, such as mammography.

ALTERNATIVES

At present, this type of bone densitometry is the most accurate. There are several ultrasound-based units in the initial offering phase, but there is some question of the reliability of tracking treatment. This is due to the fact that the ultrasound-based units measure bone density only in the heel. Treatment progress is better measured in other parts of the body, such as the elbow.

RECOMMENDATION

The recommendation is that a bone densitometry unit be purchased as soon as possible. The vendor has also offered training at no additional expense if an order is placed by day/month/year.

PROCEDURE CODES CPT (CURRENT PROCEDURAL TERMINOLOGY) OR HCPCS (HEALTH CARE PROCEDURE CODING SYSTEM)

As of January 1, 1997 (grace period to April 1, 1997), the following three codes are no longer recognized for Medicare payment:

76070—Computerized tomography, bone density study
76075—Dual energy x-ray absorptiometry (DEXA), bone density study
78350—Bone density (bone mineral content) study, single-photon absorptiometry

In their place, the following interim HCPCS codes are used to report bone mineral density studies:

00062—Peripheral skeletal bone mineral density studies (e.g., radius, wrist, heel)
00063—Central skeletal bone mineral density studies (e.g., spine, pelvis)
78351—Bone density (bone mineral content) study, dual photon absorptiometry. This is a noncovered service by Medicare.

MEDICARE INDICATIONS AND LIMITATIONS OF COVERAGE

A. Measurement of bone mass is a covered service when it is medically necessary and when it will render accurate and reliable information that can be used in making a clinical decision about the need to intervene therapeutically.

B. There are multiple methods for obtaining bone mass or bone density information. There is a significant difference in the safety, precision, and accuracy of the different methods. Based on this, Medicare coverage is limited to those that have been rated favorably in clinical studies.

   1. Methods of testing that have been found to be safe, precise, and accurate and are covered under Medicare Part B:

      a. Single-photon absorptiometry (formerly code 78350) is covered under Medicare when used in assessing changes in bone density of patients with osteodystrophy or osteoporosis when performed on the same individual at intervals of 6 to 12 months.

      b. Dual-energy x-ray absorptiometry (formerly code 76075). By definition, the code includes one or more sites. A DEXA study also includes a discussion of the procedure with the patient and a review of clinical data (e.g., patient history) and other pertinent radiologic studies; calibration and quality control (e.g., measurement of photons) of the device and assurance that anatomic markings are appropriately displayed and are in proper position; and assurance that quantitative data are valid and that interpretation of data, generation of the written report, and communication of the report to the referring physician and/or patient are complete.

c. Quantitative computed tomography (formerly code 76070). This service is covered under the new codes effective 01/01/97.

2. Methods of testing that are not covered under Medicare Part B: Dual-photon absorptiometry (CPT code 78351) is a noninvasive radiological technique that measures absorption of a dichromatic beam by bone material. This procedure is not covered under Medicare.

3. New codes (replaced interim codes)

a. Code 30062 is used to report single-photon absorptiometry studies, dual-energy absorptiometry studies, or computerized tomography on a peripheral skeletal bone. Also, photodensitometry (a noninvasive radiological procedure that attempts to assess bone mass by measuring the optical density of extremity radiographs with a photodensitometer) should be reported with this code.

b. Code 60063 is used to report single-photon absorptiometry studies, dual energy absorptiometry studies, or computerized tomography on a central skeletal bone.

c. All coverage indications and limitations listed in this policy apply to the new codes.

C. Clinical indications for the measurement of bone mass for which the measurement has been found to have diagnostic and/or therapeutic value are as follows:

1. Estrogen deficiency, such as

256.2	Post-ablative ovarian failure
256.3	Other ovarian failure
627.2	Menopausal or female climacteric states

2. Vertebral abnormalities and radiographic osteopenia

268.2	Osteomalacia
275.4	Disorders of calcium metabolism
733.00–733.09	Osteoporosis
733.13	Pathological fracture (e.g., collapse of vertebra)

3. Long-term glucocorticoid therapy, (962.0 or 995.2, with E9320, adrenal cortical steroids) such as in rheumatoid arthritis, asthma, chronic active hepatitis, chronic obstructive lung disease, and inflammatory bowel disease.

4. Endocrine disorders:

252.0	Primary asymptotic hyperparathyroidism
242.00–242.91	Hyperthyroidism
246.0	Disorders of thyrocalcitonin secretion
255.0	Cushing's syndrome

Screening tests are not covered by Medicare.

COVERED DIAGNOSIS CODES, ICD-9

Coding Guidelines and Claim Submission

1. List the ICD-9 diagnosis for the reason for the test.
2. The code description indicates that multiple sites, whether peripheral or skeletal, should be billed as one unit of service. Likewise, multiple testing methods measuring peripheral and/or skeletal bone should be billed as one unit of service.
3. Documentation supporting medical necessity including the reason for testing, the method used, and the site(s) evaluated, plus a test report should be in the patient's medical record.
4. When billing for screening tests (including tests on high-risk patients), use the ICD-9 code that represents the reason for the test: V70-V70.9, V82.8–V82.9.
5. The new interim codes have three components: global, technical, and professional.

See Graphic 13.1.

HCFA Sets Higher Rates and New Codes for DXA

THE FEDERAL REGISTER recently published new rates for Medicare reimbursement for both axial and peripheral bone densitometry scans. Effective January 1, 1998, reimbursement for scans performed on an axial bone densitometry systems rose from $121.16 to $131.34. Reimbursement for peripheral systems increased slightly from $37.57 to $40.05. These new rates, reported on January 31, supersede an earlier announcement in which reimbursement for pDXA was erroneously calculated to be $68.97. Still, this announcement by HCFA should alleviate earlier concerns and rumors that reimbursement for bone densitometry was to be lowered.

In addition to the rate changes, HCFA has replaced the temporary billing codes for peripheral and axial bone densitometry (G0062 and G0063, respectively) with permanent CPT codes. Axial DXA scans will now be billed under CPT code 76075; peripheral sites fall under CPT 76076. These new codes and increased reimbursement levels seem to indicate a bright and stable outlook for DXA in the years to come. ■

GRAPHIC 13.1 Newspaper article delineating reimbursement for DXA.

FINANCIAL ANALYSIS

A breakeven financial analysis should be performed.

STRATEGIC PLANNING

All strategic planning should start with the development of mission and vision statements.

Development of the mission statement should start with choosing a team. The team members should consist of the chief radiologist, radiology administrator, radiology supervisors, and a facility administrative representative.

When developing the statement, services, markets, values, public image, long-term goals, priorities, and service delivery should be considered.

The wording should be brief and concise—one to two sentences. Finally, the statement should be unique to the department.

Steps in Strategic Planning

- Develop vision statement
- Develop mission statement
- Develop core values
- Develop quantitative strategic goals
- Issues/problems to explore
- Questions to ask before the session
- Discuss unique selling points
- SWOT analysis
- Diagram market
- Benchmark practice
- Develop follow-up mechanism

A strategic planning session is not a whining session. The day-to-day problems of providing radiology services should take a backseat to discussion of the overall environment surrounding the business (such as pricing, changing Medicare rules, pressure from other groups that want to do their own imaging, opportunities to joint venture, etc.) and how the business plans to respond proactively to these.

Develop Vision Statement

- The vision statement includes a vivid description of the organization as it effectively carries out its operations.
- Developing a vision statement can be quick and culture-specific. Participants may use methods ranging from highly analytical and rational to highly creative and divergent.
- This is the part where time easily gets away from you.

- The vision has become more of a motivational tool, too often including highly idealistic phrasing and activities to which the organization cannot realistically aspire.
- The organization will need to define a vision of how they want the organization to look five years from now.

To create a vision of the future, you must first have the group look at the environment and the market in which the practice exists now. It allows them to leverage their strengths and to describe how they will control the factors that limit the group's success.

Develop Mission Statement

The mission statement should be simple and practical. It is a blueprint for the actions and activities of the practice and should not be mistaken for a vision statement, which deals with aspirations and values. Rather, it should define who the group is, where it practices, and what it does.

- The mission statement describes the overall purpose of the organization.
- If the organization elects to develop a vision statement before developing the mission statement, ask, "Why does the image, the vision, exist—what is its purpose?" This purpose is often the same as the mission.
- When wording the mission statement, consider the organization's products, services, markets, values, and concern for public image, and maybe priorities of activities for survival.
- Consider any changes that may be needed in wording of the mission statement because of any new suggested strategies during a recent strategic planning process.
- Ensure that wording of the mission statement provides management and employees with some order of priorities in how products and services are delivered.
- When refining the mission, a useful exercise is to add or delete a word from the mission to realize the change in scope of the mission statement and assess how concise its wording is.
- Does the mission statement include sufficient description that the statement clearly separates the mission of the organization from other organizations?
- Performance improvement is at its heart.
- Keep in mind that quality exceeds the competition.
- The statement should define a clear direction or path.
- It should have a sharp focus and not get distracted by other alternatives.
- It should have connectivity, interdependence, and synergy.
- It should have importance for all members involved.

Suggested Core Values

- Common values
- Great professional and support staff
- Strong financial results

- Capital
- Strong vision
- Growth attitude
- "Succession" organization
- "Learning" organization
- Customer focused
- Use of technology to achieve goals

Quantitative Strategic Goals

Positioning: What is the position of the organization in its markets and among its competitors? How is it perceived by target markets? How do our competitors compare with us in terms of location and accessibility, quality of care, and image/reputation?
Segmentation: What segments of the market does the organization want to attract?
Culture: What is the culture of the organization's business?
Differentiation: How does the organization differ from its competitors? What are the special skills and competencies of the organization?
Social Responsibilities: What purposes does the organization serve beyond its own survival and profitability?

Following are some questions to consider when quantifying strategic goals:

- On what basis will we be competing for patients—and how will we succeed against competitor's strengths?
- What actions will the organization be taking over the next two to three years?
- What are our milestones to measure the organization's accomplishments?
- Are the organization's locations convenient?
- Does the organization have subspecialists who are providing a service highly desired by referring physicians?
- Does the organization have a convenient outpatient center that precertifies patients?
- Does the organization's or our hospitals have contracts with payers that require them to use the organization's services?
- Does the organization have a relationship with certain practices that refer?
- How reliable and important is each referral area to the organization?
- Why does the organization believe we get patients from certain physician groups and areas of town?
- Is there any practice or hospital marketing that has an impact on patient referrals?
- How do office managers, technologists, and others fit into the picture?
- What impact does the reputation of the organization have on referrals?
- What does the hospital consider to be its primary, secondary, and tertiary markets? What population count do they have for each market?
- Does the organization line up with the organization's hospitals, or does the organization get some patients from other areas?

- Will laws encourage or discourage outpatient centers?
  - Legal counsel is often helpful in analyzing the data in light of the upcoming legislative and regulatory changes from HCFA, Stark, Medicare, fraud and abuse, and others. How will these changes affect how the practice performs?
- How will changing laws affect joint ventures with hospitals and other referring groups?

Issues and Problems to Explore

What does the organization want to look like in three years? What are the organization's priorities for the next two to three years? What resources will the organization need to accomplish these goals? How will the organization monitor progress (what are the milestones)?

- Group structure
- Governance
- Partnership and nonpartnership status
- Retirement and partial retirement options
- Productivity
- Accommodating the diverse needs within the organization
- Hospital–physician relationships
- Problematic practice-related interactions
- Reviewing and updating of practice contracts and joint venture documents, and the proactive development of practice policies, including the consequences for breaching those policies
- Other action items such as recruiting, marketing, adding to the capabilities of the business office, and pursuing new business opportunities

Questions

Some questions to ask before a planning session include the following:

- Who are the organization's customers?
- Why are patients referred to the organization currently?
- What competition does the organization have?
- What factors will affect the organization's ability to offer imaging services in the future?
- What opportunities exist in the organization's market?

Planning Session Preparation

Agenda Item: Create a vision/mission for the organization.
Pre-Work: Have a summary sheet with anticipated legal and practice changes in the future.

Agenda Item: Brainstorm unique selling points for services that the business offers.
Pre-Work: Compile a list of all radiology services that the organization offers and specifics on the organization's reputation. Also compile data on some of the business's competitors.
Agenda Item: Analyze the organization's SWOT (strengths, weaknesses, opportunities, and threats).
Pre-Work: Compile data on some of the organization's competitors, the legal changes anticipated, the organization's expenses, trends in imaging and general referral data. Determine which areas and imaging modalities pay well and which do not.
Agenda Item: Create a diagram of the organization's market.
Pre-Work: Collect referral data by physician, patient demographic data, hospital and the organization's marketing initiatives, payers by percentage of the organization's receipts, and market data from the hospital or city.
Agenda Item: Benchmark the practice.
Pre-Work: Explore data from the American College of Radiology (ACR), Medical Group Management Association (MGMA), and Radiology Business Management Association (RBMA).
Agenda Item: Create the organizational strategies.
Pre-Work: Have referral, patient, and demographic data for each anticipated initiative.
Agenda Item: Create follow-up and monitoring mechanisms.

14 Financial Management

Finance is one of the most critical areas in an imaging department. The flow of information that affects revenue generation must also be understood. For that reason, it is logical to start with information flow in and between the HIS (hospital information system) and RIS (radiology information system). In addition, Medicare and other payer entities insist on accuracy and timeliness. Some institutions do not have a RIS, but create billing and coding functions within the HIS. The important concept to understand is that there are various types of codes that must be used to record a patient procedure.

Information is entered into the imaging department's computer system when a patient is registered to have a procedure performed. The RIS/HIS system assists in matching the entry in various tables that contain different codes and other information. This information is passed electronically to the billing department, which in turn transmits to the various payers (insurance companies, etc.).

Typically the department will have a document called the *chargemaster*. This document typically contains codes, procedure descriptions (e.g., CT abdomen), and the facility's charge. This document must be constantly updated. Medicare has its own set of descriptions, and these are changed and modified on an annual basis. Medicare also adds and deletes codes annually. In some cases, temporary codes are created for new procedures. As an example, bone densitometry had a temporary code before Medicare decided to reimburse for the procedure. Initially, it had to be reported even though no reimbursement was received.

Many facilities also have what are called *internal descriptions*, which may have slightly different wording. These are for use only within the facility.

CODE DEFINITIONS

The government and other entities have established various codes to describe disease conditions, imaging procedures, and other situations. These codes, along with their definitions, are listed below.

ICD-9 CM (International Classification of Diseases, Clinical Modification) are codes that describe medical or disease condition. Example: 349.1.

CPT-4 (current procedural technology) codes were developed by the American Medical Association. They are used to describe an exam or procedure, usually a five-digit code. Other medical areas, such as lab and surgery, use CPT codes. The charge associated with a code should include the procedure and any associated supplies. Modifiers may be added to increase or reduce representation of resources. Example: 71020-TC is the CPT code for a two-view chest x-ray.

HCPCS (Health Care Administration's Common Procedural Coding System) codes were developed by Medicare as a way to build on CPT codes. They are used by local carriers (insurance companies contracted to bill for Medicare). There are several levels of codes within the HCPCS system. *Level I* codes are the same as CPT codes. *Level II* codes are nationally used and begin with the letters A through V. Local codes are *Level III* codes and begin with the letters W through Z.

Revenue codes are three-digit codes developed to categorize revenue associated with a CPT code.

NCF (national conversion factor) is a specific dollar amount and is periodically changed by the government. It is used to determine payment. When multiplied by the total of the components for one procedure, the resultant payment can be determined.

DRGs (diagnostic related groups) are used by Medicare to reimburse inpatients for procedures and services associated with a given disease condition. A set amount is paid regardless of the resources expended.

APCs (ambulatory patient classifications) are basically outpatient DRGs.

EM (evaluation and management) is coding that can be done for some imaging procedures, such as a pre-procedure history and physical.

ABN (advanced beneficiary notice) is a form (not a code) that Medicare patients sign stating they will pay the portion that Medicare does not.

RBRVS (resource-based relative value system) was developed to assign relative amounts of resources utilized for procedures performed. This is used to measure workload and also in developing payment for procedures. These codes are broken down into components:

- Physician work RVU (relative value unit)
- Practice expense RVU
- Malpractice expense RVU

The RBRVS is used in conjunction with a GPCI (geographical practice cost index), which takes into account local conditions.

The coding system is complex. Imaging procedures typically have two major components. One component is *technical* (all nonradiologist charges). It is usually listed with the modifier TC after the code. The other component is *professional* (radiologist or physician charges), which codes are usually listed with the modifier PC afterward. The codes can also have associated revenue codes, supply codes (technical), surgical procedure codes (technical), and others. Some institutions utilize global billing, which is billing for the institution and physician in one bill. These include both the PC and TC with no modifier after the CPT code. For global billing the total RVU = PC + TC.

Calculations may become very complex when Medicare adds modifiers, adjustments, and so forth. For example, what is termed a *nonfacility* is a nonhospital entity, such as an outpatient imaging center. The following components are used in the calculation:

GPCI (geographic practice cost indexes)—adjust reimbursement based on part of the country
RVU—relative value units
PE—practice expense
MP—malpractice
W—work

Refer to Graphic 14.1. For example, the formula for calculating 2008 (PC) physician fee schedule payment amount is as follows in box.

EXAMPLE

2008 Nonfacility Pricing Amount = [(Work RVU × Budget Neutrality Adjustor (0.8806)) (round product to two decimal places) × Work GPCI) + (Transitioned Nonfacility PE RVU × PE GPCI) + (MP RVU × MP GPCI)] × Conversion Factor

The resultant number is multiplied by the Medicare fee schedule amount to give what is paid. It is obvious from the example how complex the calculation system is!

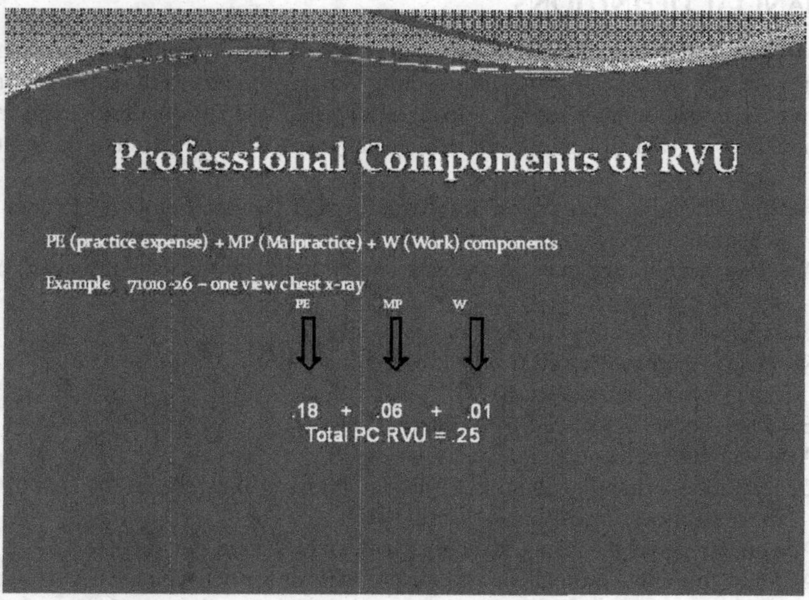

GRAPHIC 14.1 Graphic description of professional components of RVU breakdown.

Insurance entities typically follow Medicare guidelines after a while. *Precertification* (approval to perform the exam) is required by most insurance entities. ABN (advanced beneficiary notice) forms are required for Medicare patients.

It is important to stay abreast of regulation changes. As an illustration of this point, recent changes in regulations have introduced a *contiguous body part* factor, which states that when contiguous body parts are imaged during the same session (e.g., CT abdomen and pelvis), the fee paid is less than if they were imaged at separate sessions.

The Medicare fee schedule also contains RVUs for *transitions*. These are for facilities transitioning from nonacceptance of Medicare to acceptance of Medicare. Those entities who participate in the Medicare program are called *Par* (participating) and those who choose not to are called *Non-par* (nonparticipating).

Refer to Chart 14.1 for a sample Medicare fee schedule.

Codes must match when submitted. For example, the ICD-9 must match CPT, which must match revenue code, and so forth, or the submission is rejected. Documentation is the key—what is not documented *did not occur*. Everything used to bill should be in the radiologist's report. Many billing departments are now billing the PC component directly from radiologist dictation rather than codes submitted by the hospital. Additionally, many institutions are now employing radiology coders specifically trained in coding radiology procedures for payment submission.

An additional fact is that if an entity is new (such as a new MRI center, etc.), it can take several months for Medicare approvals for both the facility itself and the radiologists. This severely affects cash flow.

FINANCIAL DEFINITIONS

It is important to be familiar with financial terms, as they encompass a language of their own. The manager will be constructing various spreadsheets, as well as interpreting the information on reports. Financial terms are used to standardize this information. Below is a listing of important financial terms along with a short description.

FASB—Financial Accounting Standards Board—sets protocols for financial accounting reporting
Assets—those things that have worth; can be hard (buildings, equipment) or soft (patents)
Liabilities—things for which money is owed
Revenue—income derived from a product or service
Income—worth derived (cash)
Expense—costs associated with deriving income
APR—annual percentage rate
Depreciation—the allocation, generally monthly or annually, of the cost of a fixed asset over its estimated useful life
Accounts receivable—amounts that have been billed but not collected
Accounts payable—amounts owed for products or services received
Quick ratio—current assets divided by current liabilities
NPV—net present value

HCPCS	MOD	Description	Work RVU	Transitioned Non-FAC PE RVU	Fully Implemented Non-FAC PE RVU	Transitioned Facility PE RVU	Fully Implemented Facility PE RVU	MP RVU	Transitioned Non-Facility Total	Fully Implemented Non-Facility Total	Transitioned Facility Total	Fully Implemented Facility Total
71010		Chest x-ray	0.18	0.48	0.43	0.48	0.43	0.03	0.69	0.64	0.69	0.64
71010	TC	Chest x-ray	0.00	0.42	0.37	0.42	0.37	0.02	0.44	0.39	0.44	0.39
71010	26	Chest x-ray	0.18	0.06	0.06	0.06	0.06	0.01	0.25	0.25	0.25	0.25

CHART 14.1 Sample Medicare fee schedule. Graphic description of professional component RVU breakdown.

Amortization—repayment of a loan in installments
Annualizing—taking an amount for a certain period and calculating its value for one year
Collateral—asset that is used for assurance
IRR—internal rate of return
EBITA—earnings before interest, taxes, and amortization
Gross margin—gross revenue minus gross expense
Operating income—income from operations that does not include things such as interest from investments
Return on equity—the amount or percentage that an asset generates
Weighted average—an average that takes into account how much each component has contributed

FINANCIAL STATEMENTS

There are two common financial statements that are used to examine an entity's financial status. The first is the balance sheet. The second is the income statement.

A *balance sheet* is a financial statement that represents a financial snapshot of where the business entity is right now. It gauges the financial strength of an entity. On the statement, assets, liabilities, and remaining equity are listed in categories. *Short-term assets* are assets that are easily convertible to cash, such as cash and accounts receivable. *Accounts receivable* are services that have been performed but not collected for. *Long-term assets* are assets that consist of items such as buildings, equipment, and so forth. *Total assets* is the sum of long- and short-term assets.

Liabilities are items such as *accounts payable,* which are bills due. There are basically two types of liabilities: *Short-term liabilities* are those of relatively short duration such as short-term bank loans. Long-term liabilities are those of relatively long duration such as mortgages.

Retained equity is the owner's initial financial input plus any earnings that have been retained (owner's equity), less any payments to owners generally referred to as dividends. The basic balance sheet formula is as follows:

$$\text{assets} = \text{liabilities} + \text{retained equity}$$

The *income statement* represents an accounting of income and expenses for a given period. Two common accounting methods are used in the income statement: cash and accrual. In the *cash method,* income actually received in a given period is counted. In the *accrual method,* what is owed for that period is used, even though it may not have been collected yet. Refer to Chart 14.2 for a sample balance sheet.

There are five basic sections to an income statement:

Revenue—amount billed for the period; also called *gross billings.*
Contractual Allowances—amount allotted for reductions such as Medicare, managed care contracts, etc.
Net Revenue—revenue minus allowances.

XYZ Imaging Co.	
Statement of Financial Position (Balance Sheet)	
1-Mar-08	
Current Assets	
Cash	$100,000
Cash - Restricted (have on hand, but committed)	$25,000
Prepaid Expenses (insurance, etc.)	$15,000
Accounts receivable	$150,000
Total Current Assets	$290,000
Property and Equipment	
Computers	$80,000
CT Scanner	$890,000
MRI Scanner	$1,300,000
Total Property and Equipment	$2,270,000
Less accumulated depreciation	$(83,500)
Net Property and Equipment	$2,186,500
Total Assets	$2,476,500
Current Liabilities	
Accounts Payable	$25,000
Loans Payable	$1,800,000
Total Liabilities	$1,825,000
Owner's Equity	$651,500

CHART 14.2 Sample balance sheet.

Expenses—line item listing of expenses allocated for that period. There are a variety of ways to list expenses, depending on the business entity. Typically, items such as staff and supply costs are included. To ensure accuracy, the user must understand the accounting system used; for example, the department may have accounting for supply orders across multiple periods—ordered one month, received the next, billed the third. How the expense is allocated is the key to the truest possible statement.

Profit—net revenue minus expenses equals profit.

Most business entities pay taxes on a quarterly basis. The user must be sure that provisions are made to put aside taxes on that profit.

Refer to Chart 14.3 for a sample income statement.

FINANCIAL RATIOS

It is important to have some familiarity with the terms used to analyze these statements. *Financial ratios* are used to measure performance against *industry standards*. Definitions of some common ratios follow:

XYZ Imaging Co. Statement of Income for the Month Ended May 2008	
Revenues	**Month**
Technical Services	$220,000
Less allowances	$(105,000)
Net Revenues	$115,000
Operating Expenses	
Contracted Services	$15,000
Supplies	$890
Equipment leased	$23,000
Repairs	$8,000
Administrative fees	$2,000
Staff salaries and benefits	$35,000
Marketing	$500
Postage	$95
Total Operating Expenses	$84,485
Net Income From Operations	$30,515
Provision for taxes (33%)	$10,070
Net Income (Loss) After Taxes	$20,445

CHART 14.3 Sample income statement.

- Accounts Receivable Ratio—current accounts receivable balance divided by average monthly gross revenues.
- Gross Collection Percentage—collections divided by gross charges.
- Current Ratio—current assets divided by current liabilities.
- Debt-to-Equity Ratio—liabilities divided by equity. Ascertains financial strength.
- Return-on-Assets Ratio (ROA)—earnings before interest and taxes (EBIT) divided by net operating assets; determines what an investment (in capital equipment, etc.) is earning. For profit, this must be higher than loan interest being paid.
- Gross profit margin ratio—gross profit divided by total sales. If this is low, your prices may be too low. The converse is also true.

BUDGETING

One of the most important tasks a manager will be asked to do by upper management is to construct a budget. In simple terms, a budget is a document that plans for income and spending based on a variety of factors. Managers are expected to understand accounting and finance on a more detailed level than in the past. Depending on the institution, the finance departments may handle these functions. However, line-level managers are expected to have a basic understanding of constructing budgets and financial reporting.

There are major types of budget construction. One is *zero-based budgeting*, where historical figures are not used. The other is *historical budgeting*, which uses data from previous periods. A combination of both of these methods may also be used.

Important Considerations

Some considerations when constructing a budget should come from a well-written business plan. How much can be spent on equipment and supplies? How much staff should be utilized? The business plan gives a good overall view and the budget should flow from there.

There are two major types of budget—*operating budgets* and *capital budgets*. Operating budgets are the day-to-day projections. Capital budgets are those used for major equipment purchases.

Operating Budget

There are four major sections to a budget, for which explanations follow: volume, price, revenues, and expenses.

Volume

The first consideration for a budget should be volume projection. When projecting exam volumes, questions should be asked such as changes from one modality to another. For example, very few myleograms are now being performed. The diagnostic information can be obtained by using CT or MRI. The volumes have moved from being counted in the myelography exam totals to being counted in CT or MRI exam totals.

There are several ways to project volumes. The first is to use historical data. Straight line (total previous year divided by 12) or seasonal (month by month) forecasting can be used.

Construction of the budget should make changes to individual months based on factors impacting it, such as increased number of mammograms in October, November, and December. (October is Breast Cancer Awareness month, and mammography volumes increase dramatically and spill over into the following months.) In addition some other entities factor in, such as people using up copays and deductibles before the end of the calendar year, when they lose them.

Price

Prices need to be established for budget purposes. Price should reflect market conditions such as competitors and other factors. When considering budget implications, data from marketing and other areas should be considered.

Imaging has hundreds of CPT codes, and each has a unique price. One simple method of establishing prices for individual CPT codes is to use a single-view chest x-ray as a multiplier using RVUs (relative value units). As an example:

EXAMPLE

1-View Chest X-ray CPT 71010-TC totally transitioned nonfacility RVU = .44 Current Price $80.00

Ribs CPT 71110-TC Totally transitioned nonfacility RVU = .73

.44/80 = .73/?

Solve for ? and the Ribs CPT code price should be $132.73.

Revenue

After volumes by modality have been established, revenues can be projected. Revenues will equal price times projected volume. However, volumes for every single CPT code cannot be predicted. Although it is possible, it is unwieldy. An easier way is to project by modality—MRI, CT, general x-ray, and so forth. As an example, all of the MRI volumes will be lumped together. However, how can revenues be projected when each MRI CPT code has its own price and volume? *Weighted averaging* is the answer. By looking at how much each individual code contributed percentage-wise to the overall volume of a modality, its dollar contribution can be determined. When all of these amounts are summed, one price is determined that represents all MRI exams. Although it is not as accurate as doing each CPT code projection, it is relatively representative for budget purposes, and much easier to determine.

In the example shown in Graphic 14.2, the contribution for 71020-TC is determined by dividing the number performed (15,000) by the total number of exams performed (52,100). This code has contributed 28.79% to the total of all exams in that modality for the past year. That percentage is then multiplied by the price for that exam, and the resulting contribution of the price to the total price for that modality is determined ($85.00 × .2879 = $24.27). All of the contribution prices are added to obtain one price representing that modality.

For purposes of illustration, it is assumed from the example that $199.84 is the representative price for the general diagnostic modality. Now that this price has been established, it can be multiplied by the volume projected for each month (assuming budgeting in monthly increments) to determine projected revenue for that month and modality.

In the diagnostic area (diagnostic or general x-ray) in the weighted averaging chart, round the amount up to $200. This is then used for the price for every month. As the chart demonstrates, gross revenue for each month can be determined.

The next step in revenue projection is determining how much will remain after various deductions. Net revenue equals gross revenue minus contractual discounts. Contracted payers will have different discounts. For example, Medicare is typically 48% of billed charges. What this means is that for every dollar Medicare is billed, the entity receives only 48 cents. Another smaller payer entity may receive a 10% discount. All of these contracts and arrangements must be considered and included

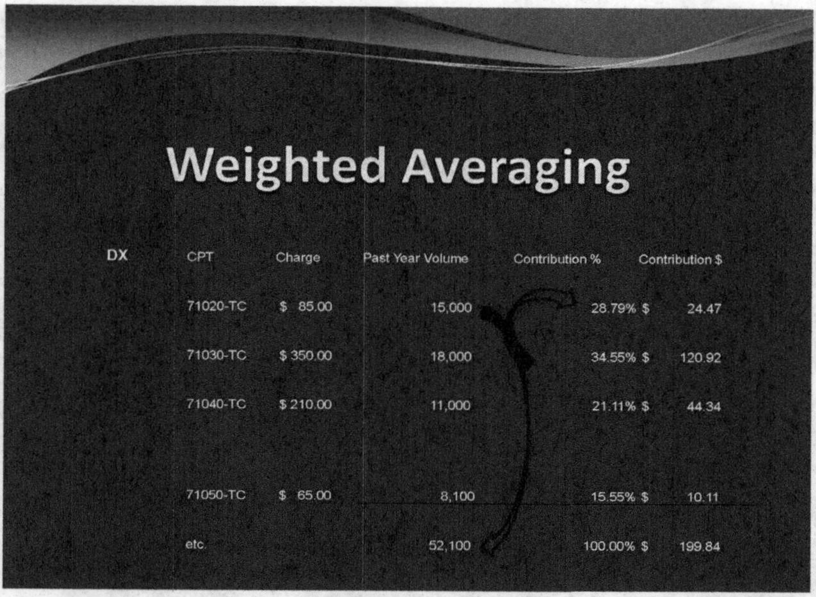

GRAPHIC 14.2 Graphic representation of weighted averaging.

in the calculation of net revenue. Again, weighted averaging can be used. The result will be one discount rate that can be applied to the gross revenues.

Other factors that must be considered are accounts sent to collection, and write-offs. Typically a small portion of what is sent to collection is never recovered. The remainder (what is not collected) is considered a write-off. The write-offs must be deducted from net revenue.

Expenses

There are two general types of expenses: *fixed expenses* and *variable expenses*. Fixed expenses do not change based on volume. Variable expenses do change with volume. Examples of variable expenses are things like barium and laundry.

For known fixed expenses in certain months, such as maintenance charges, put that amount in that particular month. For example, if it is known that an invoice for a service contract on a piece of equipment is received quarterly, that expense would be booked in March, June, September, and December.

Typically, budgets are done before the current fiscal year is over. This creates the need to *annualize*. Annualizing utilizes current year-to-date data and projects it for the entire year. Make sure to include anticipated inflation factor for those expenses that will be affected (Graphic 14.3).

Line-by-line assumptions (see Chart 14.4) should be outlined for administrative review of the budget.

Another report needed as part of the budget process is a *cash flow statement* (see Chart 14.5). This statement is created to ensure that there is enough cash to cover expenses (if not, a bank line of credit may be a consideration).

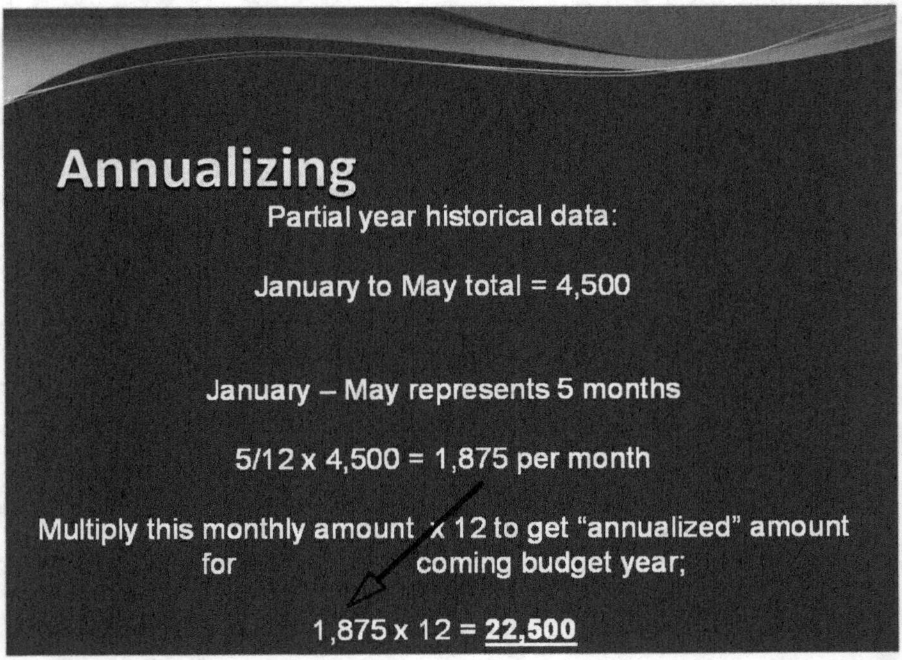

GRAPHIC 14.3 Example of annualizing.

Staffing Budget

The staffing budget should be considered separately from the general expense budget for a variety of reasons. Staffing budgets are typically done utilizing *FTE*s, or full-time equivalents. An FTE is defined by the following calculation:

$$52 \text{ weeks/year} \times 40 \text{ hours/week} = 2{,}080 \text{ hours/year}$$

The next step is to determine number of FTEs needed for basic coverage. Imaging is an on-demand business, so staffing levels cannot flex below bottom-line staffing. Support personnel must also be included—those with job titles such as file room, clerical, tech assistants, and others.

Ratios can be developed to link staffing levels to exam volumes as long as it is understood there is a floor staffing level that cannot be flexed below, and *flexible staffing* is utilized at the facility. Some facilities do not allow flex staffing.

Other factors to consider for staffing are as follows:

- Vacation hours
  - Have staff apply for vacation dates as soon as possible during the budget process so coverage can be ascertained.
- Family leave hours (if these can be anticipated)
- Lunch and break coverage

Budget Assumptions					
Revenue					
	Volumes by modality from history				
	Average charge/modality from history				
	Net revenue and net revenue % based on payer mix analysis				
Expense					
Type	**Source**				
Variable	a Can use historical or anticipated costs. In example, service contracts				
Fixed	b From past year's expenses				
Fixed	c Previous years expense/12				
Variable	d Supplies				
		YTD 200X (Jan–Dec)		$464,129	
		Jun–Dec 200X exam volume x 2		39,972	
				$11.61	/exam
			x 1.05		5% anticipated inflation factor
				$12.19	/exam
Fixed	e Previous fiscal YTD expense/12				
Fixed	f Previous fiscal YTD expense/12				
Variable	g Laundry				
		YTD 200X (Jan–Dec)		$14,000	
		Jun–Dec exam volume x 2		39,972	
				$0.35	/exam
			x 1.05		5% anticipated inflation factor
				$0.37	/exam
Fixed	h Attorneys, consultants, etc.				
Fixed	i ACR accreditation fee in November				
Variable	j Postage				
		YTD 200X (Jan–Dec)		$8,462	
		Jun–Dec 200X exam volume x 2		39,972	
				$0.21	/exam
			x .41/.37		new postal fee increase
				$0.23	/exam

CHART 14.4 Sample budget assumptions.

- Sick hours (estimate from historical)
- Special circumstances (e.g., need to "flex up" during October and November mammography months)

After all these components have been constructed, all elements are brought together into the final consolidated budget (see Charts 14.6 and 14.7; note that in

Cash Flow Analysis			
Year 1	**Month 1**	**Month 2**	**Month 3**
Projected Collections	$541,610	$541,610	$541,610
Projected Expenses			
Personnel	$5,500	$5,500	$5,500
Equipment Leases	$250,000	$250,000	$250,000
Maintenance	$5,000	$5,000	$5,000
Contract Services	$80,000	$80,000	$80,000
Operating	$114,329	$114,329	$114,329
Marketing	$500	$500	$500
Total Expenses	$455,329	$455,329	$455,329
Projected Cash			
Surplus/Deficit	$86,281	$86,281	$86,281
Cash on hand	$86,281	$172,562	$258,843

CHART 14.5 Sample cash flow analysis.

Staffing Budget			
	Rate	**Hours/month**	**$/month**
RT			
Tech 1	$25.00	173.3	$4,332.50
Tech 2	$28.00	40	$1,120.00
Tech 3	$26.00	20	$520.00
Tech 4	$27.00	30	$810.00
Tech 5	$25.00	83.3	$2,082.50
	Total hours/month	346.6	$8,865.00
	FTE/Month	2	
Clerical			
Cler 1	$15.00	90	$1,350.00
Cler 2	$13.50	83.3	$1,124.55
Cler 3	$14.00	173.3	$2,426.20
		346.6	$ 4,900.75
	FTE/Month	2	
Etc.			

CHART 14.6 Sample staffing budget.

Chart 14.7, only one-half year is shown for clarity, whereas normally the entire year is shown).

VARIANCE ANALYSIS

Variance analysis is a reporting method that compares budgeted volumes and expenses to actual volumes and expenses. It can be done monthly or for any other

Fiscal Year January – December 20XX Imaging Facility						
Consolidated Charges and Expenses						
Revenue						
	January	February	March	April	May	June
Total Exam Volumes	2,426	2,426	2,426	2,426	2,426	2,426
Gross Revenue	$1,083,220	$1,083,220	$ 1,083,220	$ 1,083,220	$1,083,220	$1,083,220
Net Revenue	$541,610	$541,610	$541,610	$541,610	$541,610	$541,610
50%						
Expenses						
Staffing	$55,000	$55,000	$55,000	$55,000	$55,000	$55,000
a Contracted Services	$80,000	$80,000	$80,000	$80,000	$80,000	$80,000
b Office Rent	$30,000	$30,000	$30,000	$30,000	$30,000	$30,000
c Equipment Leases	$250,000	$250,000	$250,000	$250,000	$250,000	$250,000
d Supplies	$29,573	$29,573	$29,573	$29,573	$29,573	$29,573
e Repairs/Maintenance	$5,000	$5,000	$5,000	$5,000	$5,000	$5,000
f Administrative Fees	$300	$300	$300	$300	$300	$300
g Laundry Costs	$898	$898	$898	$898	$898	$898
h Professional Fees	$1,000	$1,000	$1,000	$1,000	$1,000	$1,000
i Licensing/ Accreditation Costs	$0	$0	$0	$0	$0	$0
j Postage	$558	$558	$558	$558	$558	$558
k Marketing and Promotion	$500	$500	$500	$500	$500	$500
l Misc. Operating Expenses	$500	$500	$500	$500	$500	$500
n Depreciation Expense	$2,000	$2,000	$2,000	$2,000	$2,000	$2,000
	$455,329	$455,329	$455,329	$455,329	$455,329	$455,329
Net Rev – Exp.	$86,281	$86,281	$86,281	$86,281	$86,281	$86,281

CHART 14.7 Sample consolidated budget.

period needed. Variance analysis points out not only when items are not at budgeted levels, but why. There are important factors to consider.

Date of Service versus Date of Posting

Depending on the HIS/RIS/accounting systems used, the date of service when the exam was actually performed may be different than the date of posting, when the exam data is actually entered into the system. This can cause inaccurate volume counts for a particular period being considered. In addition, expenses may not actually "hit the books" when they are incurred. Something may be purchased for use during a certain month, but not actually paid for (as an expense) until later. The important thing to remember here is that the manager must ensure that expenses are allocated to the period being analyzed.

Fixed expenses are also a part of this process. By creating the variance report, the manager can ensure that they are budgeted in the correct period.

Probably more important than the period variance analysis is the year-to-date variance analysis. By looking at year-to-date data, most aberrations caused by the items previously mentioned are part of the data. This is the most accurate way of analyzing, because expenses are not always allocated to the correct period.

Certain items should not fluctuate, such as rent and service contracts.

The variance analysis should contain gross revenues (amounts billed) and net revenues (amounts actually paid or collected). It is also important to know whether the *cash* or *accrual* method of accounting is being used. The simple definition of the cash method accounts for only what has been collected. The accrual method accounts for what is owed (accounts receivable) to the entity and what the entity owes (accounts payable). Refer to Chart 14.8 for a sample variance analysis.

RETURN ON INVESTMENT

The return on investment (ROI) analysis is usually a presentation made to a CFO (chief financial officer) or CEO (chief executive officer) that demonstrates if a project will make or lose money.

Companies usually get money in two ways: *debt*, which is borrowing money, and *equity*, which is obtained through raising money through stock sales, retained earnings (profit), and so forth. Part of this consideration is the *opportunity cost*, which is the amount that other investments would have returned. In doing this analysis, the *weighted average cost of capital*—what money will cost taking the debt and equity portions of a company into account, using the proportion of each component—is used.

Weighted Average Cost of Capital Formula

$$w_d(1 - \text{Tax rate})\, r_d + w_e r_e$$

where:

w_d = debt portion

r_d = cost of debt

w_e = equity portion

r_e = cost of internal equity

The *cost of debt* is the interest percentage being paid now for borrowed money. The *cost of internal equity* is the interest that would be paid if the money (cash, retained earnings, etc.) were put in a bank or other investment.

The weighted average cost of capital, then, is the amount that the money from the debt and equity portions could earn (using the proportion of each normally employed by the company) if invested in some way other than the project that is being proposed.

Month:	Month, Year					
	Actual	Budget	Variance	YTD Actual	YTD Budget	Variance
Total Exam Volume	2,500	2,426	74	25,000	26,000	(1,000)
Gross Revenue[1]	$1,000,000	$970,400	$29,600	$ 10,000,000	$ 10,400,000	$(400,000)
Net Revenue	$475,000	$485,200	$(10,200)	$4,500,000	$5,200,000	$(700,000)
(collection %)	48%	50%		45%	50%	
Expenses	**Actual**	**Budget**	**Variance**	**YTD Actual**	**YTD Budget**	**Variance**
Staffing	$58,000	$55,000	($3,000)	$550,000	$560,000	$10,000
Contracted Services	$139,000	$130,000	($9,000)	$1,300,000	$1,331,163	$31,163
Office Rent	$46,500	$35,000	($11,500)	$385,000	$350,000	($35,000)
Equipment Leases	$210,000	$210,000	$0	$2,095,000	$2,100,000	$5,000
Supplies	$25,000	$33,000	$8,000	$309,895	$330,000	$20,105
Repairs/Maintenance	$35,000	$37,000	$2,000	$411,304	$370,000	($41,304)
Administrative Fees	$3,350	$4,450	$1,100	$44,440	$44,500	$60
Laundry Costs	$22,500	$24,500	$2,000	$259,829	$245,000	($14,829)
Professional Fees	$6,000	$5,750	($250)	$55,000	$57,500	$2,500
Licensing/ Accreditation Costs	$1,000	$800	($200)	$8,141	$8,000	($141)
Postage	$1,200	$1,500	$300	$14,850	$15,000	$150
Marketing and Promotion	$1,200	$1,150	($50)	$10,465	$11,500	$1,035
Misc. Operating Expenses	$1,100	$1,050	($50)	$ 9,850	$10,500	$650
Depreciation Expense	$13,000	$13,000	$0	$130,000	$130,000	$0
	$504,850					
Net Revenue – Expense	($29,850)					
Variable Expenses	**Bgt/Exam**	**Actual/ Exam**				
Supplies	$13.60	$10.00				
Laundry Costs	$0.33	$0.40				
FTE/Exam	0.005152514	0.00500000				

1. $400/exam budgeted

CHART 14.8 Sample variance analysis report.

The ROI calculations look at a project on strictly financial terms. You may need to upgrade or add equipment for other reasons (competition, etc.), which may not necessarily make the project a cash cow.

Some fundamentals of how money works will be examined to help understand this concept. Receiving a dollar today is worth more than receiving a dollar tomorrow (it has more time to grow).

As an example, if $1 is invested at an interest rate of 10% per year, in five years, it would be would be worth $1.61:

Year 0	Year 1	Year 2	Year 3	Year 4	Year 5
$1.00	$1.10	$1.21	$1.33	$1.46	$1.61
× 1.10%		× 1.10%		etc.	

This illustrates the concept of *compound interest.*

Net Present Value

Undertaking the time value of money is the key to understanding the next concept, which is *net present value,* or NPV. NPV shows what a dollar from a group of future periods is worth in *today's* terms. This is called *discounting,* or *discounted cash flow* (DCF).

DCF uses the cash flow from future years and states what that worth is at this moment. We take the previously described compounding process and look at it in reverse to determine what a value is today from future years.

Refer to Chart 14.9. If the DCF is positive, you are doing better than breaking even and are making money on the project. This has a positive value of $78, so the project should be undertaken.

At this point in time, use 12% in the formula as the interest rate (this is the industry average for the medical business).

The Excel formula is

NPV = (i%, value a, value b, value c …)

where i is the interest (12%, and values a … z) are the cash flows. Make sure to include the investment in year 1, which is a negative cash flow.

Simple Cash Flow Statement	Net Present Value (NPV)	Year 0	Year 1	Year 2	Year 3	Year 4
Equipment Purchase		$ (1,500)				
Income			$ 2,810	$ 3,550	$ 4,500	$ 5,750
Expenses			$ 2,500	$ 3,150	$ 4,000	$ 5,000
		$ (1,500)				
Cash			$ 310	$ 400	$ 500	$ 750
		$ 287				
$78 (Sum)		$ 343				
		$ 397				
		$ 551				
		$ 78		at 8%	(used just for example)	

CHART 14.9 Discounted cash flow sample.

Internal Rate of Return

The second way projects are usually analyzed is by using the *internal rate of return* (IRR). Using this method, the formula is basically reversed. The sum is "forced" to zero, to see what the resulting interest rate will be.

By forcing the NPV to equal 0, we determine the rate of return we are now getting from other projects. In this case, it returns 10%.

The Excel formula is

$$\text{IRR} = (\text{value a, value b, value c} \ldots)$$

where values equal cash flows. Again include negative cash flow in year 1.

A *sensitivity analysis* (Chart 14.10) is looking at different results after changing anything that is variable to see if the project is still viable.

Try different variables that could realistically happen (see Charts 14.11, 14.12, and 14.13). Analyze the results to make the decision.

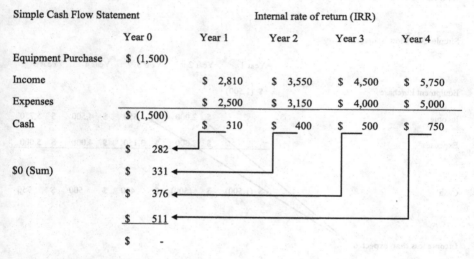

Simple Cash Flow Statement **Internal rate of return (IRR)**

	Year 0	Year 1	Year 2	Year 3	Year 4
Equipment Purchase	$ (1,500)				
Income		$ 2,810	$ 3,550	$ 4,500	$ 5,750
Expenses		$ 2,500	$ 3,150	$ 4,000	$ 5,000
Cash	$ (1,500)	$ 310	$ 400	$ 500	$ 750
	$ 282 ← (Year 1)				
$0 (Sum)	$ 331 ← (Year 2)				
	$ 376 ← (Year 3)				
	$ 511 ← (Year 4)				
	$ -				

CHART 14.10 Sensitivity analysis.

Simple Cash Flow Statement

	Year 1	Year 2	Year 3	Year 4	Year 5
Equipment Purchase	$(1,500)				
Income		$2,810	$3,550	$4,500	$5,750
Expenses		$2,500	$3,150	$4,000	$5,000
Cash	$(1,500)	$310	$400	$500	$750
changing from 8% to 12% interest					
NPV	$(64)				

CHART 14.11 Sample cash flow statement.

Simple Cash Flow Statement

	Year 1	Year 2	Year 3	Year 4	Year 5
Equipment Purchase	$ (1,500)				
Income		$ 2,810	$ 3,550	$ 4,500	$ 5,750
Expenses		$ 2,900	$ 3,300	$ 4,000	$ 5,000
Cash	$ (1,500)	$ (90)	$ 250	$ 500	$ 750

Expenses higher than expected **NPV** **$ (390)**

CHART 14.12 Sensitivity analysis sample.

Simple Cash Flow Statement

	Year 1	Year 2	Year 3	Year 4	Year 5
Equipment Purchase	$ (1,500)				
Income		$ 2,000	$ 3,550	$ 4,500	$ 5,750
Expenses		$ 2,500	$ 3,150	$ 4,000	$ 5,000
Cash	$ (1,500)	$ (500)	$ 400	$ 500	$ 750

Income less than expected

NPV **$ (622)**

CHART 14.13 Result if income is not what is expected.

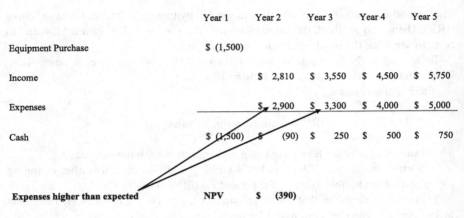

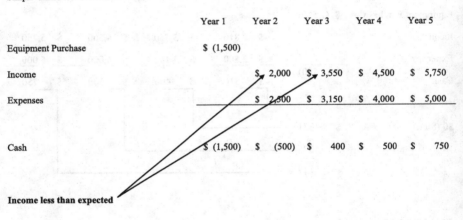

15 Capital Equipment

CONSIDERATIONS

Capital equipment has different definitions, depending on the accounting treatment. Typically, it refers to equipment over $5,000 in acquisition cost.

Major considerations must be made when purchasing or leasing capital equipment: *replacement* for existing technology, *upgrade* of existing technology, *new* technology, and equipment at the end or past its *useful life*. Additional considerations are return on investment, competitive advantage, changes in demographics fueling increased or decreased use, and the utilization of loss leaders.

Replacement usually occurs when equipment has become aged or cannot be used for some other reason. Many times, equipment can be upgraded to existing technology by replacing software or hardware. Refurbished equipment is also an option, and it is typically much cheaper than new equipment.

New technology can also fuel the need to buy capital equipment. This is usually driven by competition or demand from the public. A recent example is digital mammography. When the advantages of this technology were learned by the public, patients started to inquire if it was available when calling for appointments.

Equipment should be replaced when it reaches the end of its useful life. This varies by use and modality. For example, a standard radiographic room may last for many years, as the technology does not change much. A four-slice computed tomography (CT) scanner is still relevant even though there are scanners up to 320 slices at the time of this publication. If a piece of equipment is used only casually, it will usually outlive its published useful life. Most vendors will supply useful life charts if requested.

A loss leader is a program or service offered that does not generate a profit but usually results in spin-off business that is profitable. A good example is screening mammography. To be competitive, screening mammograms are offered at a prices that many times does not cover the cost of the exam. However, mammography results in breast biopsies and other procedures that typically are profitable.

It is helpful to utilize a replacement plan. The horizon can be any number of years, but five years is typically used. A sample is shown in Table 15.1.

CAPITAL ACQUISITION AND PLANNING TEAM

Because imaging-related equipment is usually very expensive, it is considered to have a very high *acquisition cost*. A business plan must justify replacement or an initial purchase. The *capital acquisition team* should consist of the following members:

- Radiologist "champion"
- Radiology administrator

TABLE 15.1
Sample Five-Year Replacement Plan

Model	Age	Hours/ Week	Estimated Useful Life	Location	Volume 5-Yr Market Growth %	Projected Volume Growth	Service Costs Last 2 Years	Software Level	Equipment Condition (1–5 Scale)	Utilization %	Future Technology	Comments
C-arm	7	28	10									
C-arm	1	21	10									
Portable #1	17	35	10									
Portable #2	12	35	10									
Laser Printer	9	24/7	5	workroom								
Room 1	8	42	10	Rm 1								
Room 2	8	18	10	Rm 2								
Room 3	3	84	7	Rm 3								
Broker	0	24/7	5									
CD Burner	0	200/mo.	5	workroom								
Digital	1		5	Mam 1								
Stereo Table 5		7	Mam 2									
Biopsy Device	5		7	Mam 3								
Digital Workstation/ Software	1			Rad reading								
Mammo Tracking Software				Mam 3								
US 1	3	70	7	US 1								
US 2	3	55	7	US 2								
Nuc Room	9		12	Nuc								
Film Scanner	6 mo.	24/7	5	workroom								

PACS System	2	24/7	see comments		upgrade in 5 years
CT Scanner	0		7	CT	
Patient Monitor	11				
Hi Speed	10		15	MR	
Injector	10		15	MR	
Patient Monitor	10			MR	
CR Reader 1	2	24/7	5	workroom	
CR Reader 2	2	24/7		workroom	
160 kVA UPS		24/7	3	MR	battery replacement 20XX
100 kVA UPS	0	24/7		CT	

- Facilities representative
- Finance representative
- IT representative
- Biomed representative
- Purchasing department representative

Input should be solicited from technologists using the equipment. The capital plan should be part of the overall department and facility strategic plan.

BUDGETING FOR CAPITAL ACQUISITION

While the equipment is being replaced or installed, monies must be budgeted for equipment rental (e.g., mobile unit) if necessary.

The next decision should be if the equipment will be leased or bought outright.

The decision to lease results in no large up-front cash outlay. Cash flow typically covers the lease payment. There is no depreciation to track and allocate. Typically, there is an option to buy at end of lease. Leasing also involves certain considerations:

Major advantage—allows flexibility with quickly changing technology, upgrades during life of asset, etc.

Disadvantage—cash outlay over life of asset is more than outright buying if purchase option exercised

Buying

Buying equipment usually means a high upfront cash outlay. Also, deprecation can affect the balance sheet, misrepresenting a company's financial position. A question that also must be answered is whether the asset will produce more profit than if the same amount of cash was invested some other way.

Capital versus Operating Lease

There are two common types of lease agreements: a *capital lease* and an *operating lease*. The capital lease is tracked separately from a normal operating budget. Typically, a facility has financial "floor" for a capital lease. This means that a capital lease will not be considered for equipment cost below a certain amount. This decision depends on the company's accounting practices.

The operating lease is considered part of the normal operating budget.

The exam volume needed for when net revenue minus net expenses equals the amount paid for equipment is part of the determination of breakeven analysis. This is easier to understand graphically (see Graph 15.1).

Breakeven Analysis

As part of capital planning, a *breakeven analysis* is performed. This determines how many procedures need to be done to pay for the equipment and associated expenses.

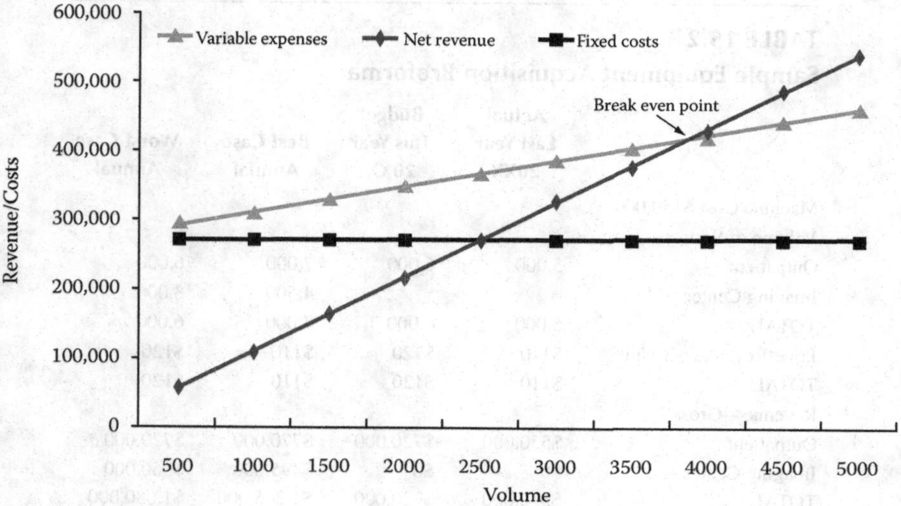

GRAPH 15.1 Graphic repesentation of breakeven analysis.

The breakeven point is defined as the exam volume at which net revenues equal fixed plus variable expenses. Components are as follows:

- Charge/exam
- Volume
- Deductions from revenue
- Expected discounts, Medicare, etc.
- Net revenue
- Direct expenses
- Indirect expenses
- Overhead, depreciation, etc.

See Table 15.2.

VENDOR RELATIONSHIPS

An important aspect not to be overlooked when considering the purchase of equipment are the vendors. Familiarize yourself with who the "players" are in each modality. These relationships can be very beneficial. Many times vendors have software to help with breakeven analyses and so forth. However, the purchaser must also beware that the analysis may be unrealistically slanted toward profit.

Vendors usually supply education and can be a great resource for learning. In addition, they can supply marketing materials that are very well done. Large vendor companies have large research and development departments that can do analyses much better than an individual (demographic changes, etc.). This analysis is vital in projecting exam volumes based on patient age, demographics, and other factors. Try

TABLE 15.2
Sample Equipment Acquisition Proforma

	Actual Last Year 20XX	Budget This Year 20XX	Best Case Annual	Worst Case Annual
Machine Cost $150,000				
Volume of Services				
Outpatient	5,000	6,000	7,000	6,000
Imaging Center			4,500	3,000
TOTAL	5,000	6,000	7,000	6,000
Price/Revenue per Unit	$110	$120	$110	$120
TOTAL	$110	$120	$110	$120
Revenue—Gross				
Outpatient	$550,000	$720,000	$770,000	$720,000
Imaging Center	$0	$0	$495,000	$360,000
TOTAL	$550,000	$720,000	$1,265,000	$1,080,000
Deductions from Revenue				
–40.00%				
Combined	$220,000	$288,000	$506,000	$432,000
NET REVENUE	$330,000	$432,000	$759,000	$648,000

to view vendor-provided information as generically as possible. The imaging manager must be aware of political ramifications—such as large manufacturers that are based locally may have a greater influence on decision making—especially when it comes to how much input upper administration has in the purchase decision. They may have political affiliations that can affect the decision.

Some other sources of background research include talking to peers about different vendors and salespersons. A visit with RSNA (Radiologic Society of North America) to get to know who makes what and who is considered cutting edge in that modality is most helpful. The RSNA annual meeting in the fall is the largest medical imaging vendor congregation in the world.

REQUEST FOR PROPOSAL

A request for proposal (RFP) is a comprehensive document that states all of the purchaser's needs and asks probing questions about the equipment being considered. The document is designed with questions that enable the purchaser to compare and rank responses among different vendors. For the most complete analysis, the purchaser must supply necessary statistics and data: volumes, types of procedures to be performed, and so forth. Second, list required and optional components and features. A medical physicist should be utilized to formulate specifications.

Make sure the RFP is specific to the piece of equipment being considered. Request the vendor company background to assess long-term viability. Many equipment companies have come and gone. It would be a mistake to purchase a large capital item from a company that might not be around in a few years.

Conduct site visits for final candidates. Discuss the performance of the equipment and the company. Talk to the administrators, radiologists, and technologists using the equipment.

When the final analysis is to be done, specify the criteria and the weighting scale. Also request the following:

- Delivery
- Installation (facility modification costs and build outs)
- Acceptance testing
- Remedies if what is promised is not delivered
- Training
- Guaranteed uptime (in most cases 98–99%)
- Availability of parts
- Guaranteed response time with penalties for noncompliance
- Warranty
- Marketing assistance if applicable
- Clearly defined upgrade path and associated costs (software upgrades, etc.)
- Ancillary equipment options and costs
- State payment terms, typically 10% with the order, 80% on delivery, and 10% on first use after successful acceptance testing

Use outside resources that specialize in helping to purchase and analyze equipment and companies, such as MDBuyline.

ACCEPTANCE/PERFORMANCE TESTING

Acceptance testing should be performed after installation and training has been completed. Equipment should not be accepted until these tests are passed. Typically, payment is then made upon the first clinical use.

Reasons for acceptance testing include the following:

- Testing ensures value (getting what you paid for).
- Standard quality tests should be conducted.
- Tests are specific to modality.
- State and federal regulations should be satisfied.
- Radiation production, scanner, magnetic fields, and so forth are dependent on modality.

A medical physicist should be employed for this process.

SERVICE CONTRACTS AND OPTIONS

Service contracts should be negotiated at purchase time if possible. Many times the vendor will bundle in multiyear discounts if the service is purchased or contracted for at the time of the sale. An extended warranty should be negotiated if possible.

Warranty start time should be determined: after install or after first clinical use. The buyer should also demand that the warranty be extended beyond expiration date by number of days/hours unit is down.

Service Contract Components

- Typical cost is 10% to 15% of purchase price.
- Training for in-house personnel should be included (biomed training).
- Response time should be delineated.
- Are upgrades—software, remote diagnostics, etc.—included or charged?
- What is the guaranteed uptime (typically 97% or better)?
- Does the contract include glassware (tubes, intensifiers, etc.)? If full coverage is not offered, glassware coverage should be prorated, at a minimum. For example, if a CT tube is warranted for 100,000 slices and goes out at 50,000 slices, the customer would only have to pay 50% of the tube replacement.
- What is the parts availability?
- Are generic parts acceptable?
- What are the after-hours charges, if any?
- What are the weekend charges?

Preventive maintenance, or PM, should be a part of any service program. PM visits are contracted for at the time the service agreement is negotiated. Following are some points to be clarified:

- How often will PM be performed?
- When are they performed (after-hours or weekends if possible)?

Types of Service Contract Options

- Original equipment manufacturer (OEM vendor).
- In-house: This is a person who works for the same institution as the imaging manager but has been trained to repair the equipment.
- Outsourced (time and materials): In this arrangement, the facility is billed for parts and labor.
- Secondary insurance: Some companies offer insurance that covers the repair of the equipment.
- Combination of any of the above, including multiple vendors.

One of the advantages of outsourcing is that the costs for repair are known. A fee is paid and all service and repair is covered. A disadvantage of outsourcing is that the

OEM may categorize these service requests as second-tier priority after their OEM customers are taken care of.

When using multiple vendors, one may not know what the other has done (service history communication).

Service Contract Rules of Thumb

- Get references.
- Contract for as long a term as possible.

Remember: Downtime = lost revenue and possible permanent disruptions to referral patterns!

Section IV

Marketing

16 Marketing

Marketing many times becomes confused with *sales*. Marketing actually defines efforts to get your product message out and influence buying, whereas sales is "closing the deal."

The first step to developing a marketing plan is to define the institution's *marketing strategy*. These three questions need to be answered:

- Where are we now?
- Where do we want to be in a year, two years, five years?
- Who do we want to be? (This comes from the strategic plan.)

The next step is to develop the *marketing plan*. Then two more questions need to be answered:

- How we will accomplish our strategy?
- What tools and methods will be used?

As a baseline, the marketing budget is usually 5% to 10% of gross sales.

An effective, successful marketing plan should follow the PDCA format: Plan, Do, Check, Act.

MEGA ISSUES

Imaging demand is projected to grow immensely in the coming years. This is due to a number of factors such as the aging population, increased Medicare population, increased advances in imaging with examples such as positron emission tomography (PET), vertebroplasty, computerized angiography (CTA), colonography, coronary magnetic resonance angiography (coronary MRA), molecular imaging, and others.

TRENDS

The government via CMS (Center for Medicare and Medicaid Services) and other payers are putting increasing scrutiny on imaging procedures. They are consistently looking for ways to decrease utilization, price, or both.

There is also a corresponding increase in credentialing (American Imaging Management [AIM], Intersocietal Commission for Accreditation of Nuclear Laboratories [ICANL], etc.) entities to ensure quality. An increase in precertification or preauthorization is occurring and will continue to accelerate in the future.

Referring offices demand the latest technology. They want to be able to order electronically and receive results electronically. They also want to be able to see actual studies via the picture archiving and communication system (PACS). Imaging entities that do not have these capabilities will lag behind or go out of business.

To complicate this scenario, decreased useful life due to technology changes results in decreased return on investment by making the life of depreciation shorter.

The Deficit Reduction Act of 2005, as well as other current legislation, is aimed in part squarely at imaging. The results are a decrease in Medicare payments, which is usually followed by a decrease in payments of private payers. There are entities in existence doing imaging exams 24/7!

It is obvious that very careful and diligent planning must be done in order to be successful.

BASIC TENETS OF MARKETING

The basic building blocks of marketing are *price, product, place,* and *promotion.*

Price

Where does the entity want to be? Since quality must be a given in order to compete, the following decisions must be considered:

- High quality, high price?
- High quality, medium price?
- High quality, low price?

A thorough business plan should be constructed with all three scenarios.

Product

In most cases, the *report* is the product, not the exam. As part of this product, the radiologist's willingness and ability to refer is crucial.

The business then must decide if it plans to be a full-service line or specialized. Full service would consist of all or most modalities: x-ray, CT, MRI, ultrasound, mammography. Specialty centers would have an emphasis such as a mammography center or outpatient MRI center.

Place

The third aspect that must be considered for the imaging business, place, includes considerations such as one or multiple locations, extended hours, high- or low-traffic area, suburban or urban area, and others.

Reports can be found on the Internet or from specialty services that contain demographics such as population density, age, median income, and so forth. Vendors may also have this information available.

Promotion

When deciding on an imaging marketing plan, the *target audience* must be chosen. This can be the general public or a specific segment of the public, as well as referring physicians and their *offices.* Many times the referring physicians will instruct their staff to order a certain exam and leave it up to the staff to book it. Good relationships with referring office staff are paramount. Can they get their exams scheduled in a timely manner? Are the hours the patients can have the exam performed convenient? As stated earlier, quality is a given. Lastly, how fast can accurate results be obtained? If the results are lost in a fax machine somewhere, it will not take long before the referring office votes with their feet.

Some imaging businesses have monthly breakfasts or luncheons with referring office staff to discuss issues. These can be used as a very good promotional tool.

COMPONENTS

The first component of a marketing plan is to define the product or service description. In imaging, this should be done by modality. For example, the CT scan department may be viewed as a *service line.*

The next task to be performed is to conduct an *environmental scan.* This is performed to analyze competition. This could be considered another hospital imaging department in the service area or outpatient imaging centers. What are their strengths and weaknesses? Do they have specialty areas (women's imaging, etc.)? What are they known for? What demographic do they capture? A tactic that sometimes helps in gathering this information is a *secret shopper.* For example, a woman can call an imaging center and ask: How long will it take to get an appointment? How much for a mammogram? When will my doctor get the results?

There are two basic types of marketing: internal, such as other departments in a hospital; and external, such as referring physicians' offices. Other places to market services are health and business coalitions or directly to businesses that can send patients your way.

Objectives must then be defined. What is to be accomplished? For example, increase in CT referrals, or recapture of previously lost business may be targeted.

Implementation Plan

After the objectives have been defined, an implementation plan should be developed. This should include feedback of effectiveness and outcomes, and follow-up and action on results.

Market Position

The imaging entity must decide where it wants to *position* itself. What does it want to become known for? Does it want to be the leader in MRI, for example?

Some service lines are known as *loss leaders.* Mammography is a good example. Loss leaders are not large revenue producers and may not break even, but they spawn downstream-related business—such as breast ultrasound, biopsy, or other services.

Important Questions

Some important questions must be asked and answered before embarking on a marketing campaign:

- Are there new offices/specialties to your market area?
- Is the radiologist champion leaving the practice or retiring?
- Is the entity considering addition/upgrade/deletion of a modality?
- Are reimbursement issues affecting volumes (no Medicare reimbursement for certain exam types, etc.)?
- Is there a change in case mix?
- Is capacity available? Do you need to add equipment?

It is important at this point to conduct a SWOT analysis (strengths, weaknesses, opportunities, threats) of your current business.

Referring offices look for—

- Ease of scheduling
- Registration process
- Access to radiologists
- Prompt report delivery
- Quality, cost, outcomes
- Other considerations

Quality reports delivered quickly and a good patient experience are the *minimum* to compete.

Advertising

Part of any marketing plan should include *advertising.* The components should include a department/facility background, position of the facility, and anything that makes the entity/department stand out against the competition.

Some channels of advertising include the following:

- Direct mail
- Advertising
    - Local paper
    - Professional journals
- Website

Websites are particularly important. Do *not* skimp in this area. Most patients and referring physician offices utilize websites heavily to gather information and make decisions.

A properly prepared and implemented marketing plan will aid immensely in the bottom line of any imaging endeavor.

Epilogue

As stated in the Preface, this book is not meant to be a comprehensive resource. However, the new imaging manager must be cognizant of all aspects of managing the department. Some chapters, such as Chapter 14, "Financial Management," are more thorough than others. This is because imaging departments in most institutions and outpatient centers are money makers. In many hospitals, other services could not be offered to the community if they were not subsidized by the revenues generated in medical imaging. Because of this fact, most hiring managers will expect the imaging manager to be well versed in finance.

This book gives examples of some forms, procedures, and policies required in an imaging department or outpatient imaging center. Each department or center will be different, which will require modification of these examples. Many, many resources are available in the public and private domains.

The new manager's day will not be linear and planned. The manager will have drop-in visitors, fires to put out, emergencies, staff calling in sick, tardy employees, and a wide variety of other issues to deal with.

The best advice I can give is to be flexible, keep an open mind, and keep learning. Imaging management can be a fulfilling, exciting career. Enjoy the journey!

Index

C

Printed in the United States
by Baker & Taylor Publisher Services